Paleo Diet

50 Recipes To Lose 10 Pounds The First Month

The Ultimate Paleo Meal Plan For Weight Loss Guaranteed

Luca Bucciarelli

Table of Contents

Introduction

If you're looking for help in making some healthy changes in your life and losing weight, this is the right place to be. We all know what a big role food and our eating habits play in our lives. It makes a huge difference in how your body looks, feels and functions as well. Once you notice where you've been going wrong, you need to start looking at how you can get it right and this is where we come in. Stop following fads and diets that don't work. Nothing that claims to work in a week and make any drastic changes in your body in a short while is actually healthy or effective. Learn more about what actually helps you and will work for your body. The right changes need to be implemented over a longer period of time for long lasting effects. We will tell you of one such effective method that you will swear by over time.

The focus of this book is the Paleo diet that has worked for so many people all over the world. You have probably heard of it but we will explain it further here and tell you how you can implement it. The Paleo diet is all about eating the right food and in the right manner. As you read on you will see what it is about and how it will benefit your body. Once you start following the Paleo diet you will also see a steady loss in all that unwanted weight that you had gained over a period of time. The recipes we've put together will help guide you and also make sure that you eat some delicious yet healthy meals every day.

Chapter 1: What Is The Paleo Diet And How Does It Benefit Your Body?

Like we mentioned before, this book is all about the Paleo diet. What is the Paleo diet, you ask? Well, you may have heard of it as the caveman or Stone Age diet as well. The Paleolithic diet is based on the concept of eating food that our ancestors from the caveman days would have eaten. It emphasizes that although a lot of time has passed, our bodies and genetic have not yet adapted to the food of modern times. This is why the healthier choice for your body would be to eat only what food they ate during Paleolithic times. No matter what the explanation is, once you read more about the diet, you will see that the food that is acceptable under this diet is obviously healthier than the other things we normally force into our bodies.

The Paleo diet helps you cut out unhealthy modern foods that are full of trans fats, sugars and other additive that do not benefit the body. Instead, you will be eating natural foods that are nutritious and help your body stay lean while you feel energetic the whole day. Typically, the foods will include vegetables, nuts, fruit, meats, and roots and exclude anything like dairy products, sugars, refined or processed oils, etc.

As mentioned above, you can only eat things that would have been available for consumption during Paleolithic days. Anything else is off limits.

Foods that are allowed on the Paleo diet:

Beverages include water, tea, almond or coconut milk.

Fish that hasn't been reared from the fisheries. For example, bass, salmon, tuna, trout, mackerel, halibut, etc.

Oils that are not processed like natural olive oil or coconut oil, avocado oil and macadamia oil.

Omega-3 rich eggs.

Grass fed animal meat and not meat from animals that have not been grain fed.

Nuts, as well as seeds, are allowed. Eat nuts like almonds, cashews, hazelnut, pecans, pine nuts, walnuts, etc. Seeds of sunflower or pumpkin are good.

Fresh vegetables should be eaten and cooking should be avoided as much as possible especially using processed oils. Eat a lot of spinach, asparagus, parsley, broccoli, carrots, celery, avocado, eggplants, etc. Eat starchy vegetables like yam, beets and butternut squash in moderation.

Fresh fruits but not too much of those with a high content of sugar. Anything like apple, papaya, grapes, lychee, lime, oranges, lemon, etc is good for you.

Food not allowed on the Paleo diet:

Let us look at the food that you should not be eating on the Paleo diet. It might be tough to cut it all off at once but it will get easier after the first few weeks and you will see the difference it makes.

Dairy like butter, whole milk, cheese cottage cheese, yogurt, pudding, creamer, ice cream, etc is not allowed.

Avoid soft drinks like coke, sprite, etc.

Fruit juices are also not allowed due to high sugar content but the raw fruit can be eaten.

Grains are not allowed. No corn, corn syrup, cereals, bread, oatmeal, toast, crackers, beer, pasta or anything that is made from grains.

Legumes are also off the list. No beans like black beans, fava beans, mung beans, red bean, string beans or any beans for that matter. Peas are also not allowed. No peanuts, soybean, tofu, lentil or miso either.

Artificial sweeteners are not permitted in the list either.

No meat from grain fed animals.

No snacks like fries, pretzels, chips, cookies, pastries, etc.

Avoid starchy vegetables like potato, yam, beets, yucca, etc.

No alcohol is allowed.

No energy drinks like red bull, vault, etc.

No sweets like candy bars or any chocolate products like M&M's.

You can see the difference between Paleo friendly foods and others quite clearly from the above lists. Use them as a guide to throw out any unhealthy food from your kitchen and stock up on the good stuff to help you avoid temptation.

Benefits of the Paleo diet:

You might not yet be convinced enough to go through with the Pale diet. However, once we tell you of all the benefits that you would reap, you will surely be on board. You don't need to follow this diet blindly jut because we say you should. Here, we will inform you about how you will benefit from going Paleo and you'll convince yourself to make this healthy lifestyle shift for your own well being.

The diet makes you choose healthy lean meat that will provide your body with more muscle and less fat. The anabolic protein from meat will help your body build more muscle mass that in turn promotes better metabolism. Muscle cells will be using more energy instead of being stored in fat cells.

Your gut will thank you for going Paleo. The processed food that we normally consume can cause inflammation in the stomach or intestines. Once you cut these out, your digestive tract works much better.

The anti-inflammatory foods in the Paleo diet are beneficial in preventing inflammation in your body. Paleo increases the anti-oxidants as well as phytonutrients that you consume. These help in preventing as well as healing diseases that you might otherwise suffer from.

You get a healthier balance of saturated and non-saturated fat that helps your cells to function optimally.

If you cut out unhealthy food from your diet, your body will work better all day and get naturally tired at night. This helps you get a restful night of sleep. You will notice how you start sleeping earlier and waking early as well.

Digesting and absorbing Paleo food is easier for the body and healthier as well.

You do not need to count calories for every bite that you eat. Paleo is definitely not about calorie counting and eating tiny portions that will leave you hungry.

Your energy levels are higher throughout the day without the aid of any energy drinks or countless cups of coffee. The right diet gives you sufficient energy to do what you need and get a good night's sleep. Your body will thank you for it.

The diet will help you lose a lot of weight in a healthy way. You will notice how many carbs you cut out by only eating food that is permitted on the diet.

Blood glucose levels in the body are more balanced once you cut off refined sugars and anything that spikes the levels in your blood. This is definitely helpful to deal with diabetes.

The diet helps you feel full for a longer time and avoid cravings that are untimely. Unlike other fads which tell you to eat tiny amounts of food which will ultimately make you cave in and eat more, here you eat enough to sustain you throughout the day. You can eat every meal; the difference is that the healthy food will help you feel satiated.

Your body will thank you for cutting off the fast foods that the modern diet is full of. These are barely nutritious if at all and instead harm your body in more ways than one. You also gain a lot of weight in a shorter period of time if you eat more fast food. Going Paleo helps you prevent this. Fast food is especially bad when it concerns the heart and is a major factor in obesity.

Paleo saves a lot of time and makes your meals simpler. You don't need to put much effort into Paleo meals and it isn't as complicated to think about what you need to prepare for the next meal. The food is simple and fulfilling.

You increase the amount of healthy fats in your diet and cut out unhealthy fat. The plan will ensure that you get the right amount and if you do get hungry untimely, eat what you want as long as it is Paleo approved.

Eating the right kind of food does more than half the work for you. If you want to lose weight, you need to control your cravings for food that are unhealthy. Make the right choice and eat the good kind of food that tastes better and will also keep you full. You don't need to starve yourself to lose weight. Eating Paleo will ensure that the food you eat helps you lose unhealthy fat and gain healthy muscle mass. If you add some regular exercise and healthy habits into your routine, you will see the massive turn that your body and life takes.

The Paleo diet will help you lose weight for the long haul and not just a few pounds that you gain back as soon as you usually do by following fad diets. The changes you make will benefit you for the rest of your life and living healthy will become a habit. You will look better, feel better and do everything you do much better as well. So go Paleo and see the difference.

Chapter 2: 15 Day Meal Plan

DAYS	BREAKFAST	LUNCH	SNACK	DINNER	DESSERTS
Day 1	Breakfast - Bacon and Sweet Potato Skillet	Lunch - One Dish Fish and Veggie Bake	Snack - Cajun Cauliflower Mini Dogs	Dinner - Easy Chicken Broccoli Casserole	Desserts - Apple, Almond & Blackberry Cake
Day 2	Breakfast – Paleo Breakfast Pie	Lunch - Paleo Lasagna	Snack - Buffalo Chicken Peppers	Dinner - Baked Eggplant with Tomato Thyme Salsa	Desserts - Pumpkin Pie Ice cream
Day 3	Breakfast - Paleo Blueberry Muffins	Lunch - Ground Pork Tacos	Snack - Zucchini Pasta / Noodles	Dinner - Jordanian Roast Lamb with Tahini Sauce	Desserts - Citrus Pomegranate Fruit Salad
Day 4	Breakfast - Savory Casserole	Lunch - Sichuan Style Shrimp	Snack - Bacon braised kale	Dinner - Salisbury Steak with Mushroom Gravy	Desserts - Healthy Sundae

Day 5	Breakfast - Banana Bread French toast	Lunch - Paleo Spaghetti Squash Hawaiian Pizza Pie	Snack - Deviled Eggs	Dinner - Irish Style Shepherd's Pie	Desserts - Paleo Chocolate Mousse
Day 6	Breakfast - Arugula and Leek Frittata	Lunch - Zucchini Pasta Bolognese	Snack - Chicken Fingers	Dinner - Bottle gourd with Tomatoes	Desserts - Mixed fruit Cobbler
Day 7	Breakfast - Chorizo Mashed Yam	Lunch - Pan grilled Lamb Chops and Cardoons	Snack - Mashed Sweet Potatoes	Dinner - Sesame – Ginger Chicken	Desserts - Flourless Peanut Butter Brownie Cookies
Day 8	Breakfast - Tomato Frittata	Lunch - Roasted Chicken Legs with Vegetables	Snack - Zucchini Fritters	Dinner - Paleo Lasagna	Desserts - Coconut Banana Foster
Day 9	Breakfast - Smoky Pork Carnitas	Lunch - Zucchini Pasta Bolognese	Snack - Meat Bagel	Dinner - Sesame – Ginger Chicken	Desserts - Poached Pears
Day 10	Breakfast - Breakfast Pie	Lunch - Slow-Cooker Pepper Steak	Snack - Buffalo Chicken Peppers	Dinner - One Dish Fish and Veggie Bake	Desserts - Carrot pudding

Day 11	Breakfast - Breakfast Meatballs	Lunch - Ratatouille (Vegan)	Snack - Zucchini Pasta / Noodles	Dinner - Salisbury Steak with Mushroom Gravy	Desserts - Citrus Pomegranate Fruit Salad
Day 12	Breakfast – Paleo Breakfast Pie	Lunch - Chicken Adobo	Snack - Cajun Cauliflower Mini Dogs	Dinner - Ground Pork Tacos	Desserts - Apple, Almond & Blackberry Cake
Day 13	Breakfast - Bacon and Sweet Potato Skillet	Lunch - Easy Chicken Broccoli Casserole	Snack - Paleo Nachos	Dinner - Carrots and Rutabaga Mash	Desserts - Paleo Chocolate Mousse
Day 14	Breakfast - Banana Bread French toast	Lunch - Pan grilled Lamb Chops and Cardoons	Snack - Chicken Fingers	Dinner - Paleo Spaghetti Squash Hawaiian Pizza Pie	Desserts - Pumpkin Pie Ice cream
Day 15	Breakfast - Chorizo Mashed Yam	Lunch - Sausage and Cauliflower Bake	Snack - Zucchini Fritters	Dinner - Roasted Chicken Legs with Vegetables	Desserts - Coconut Banana Foster

Chapter 3: Breakfast Recipes

Sweet Potato Breakfast Skillet with Bacon

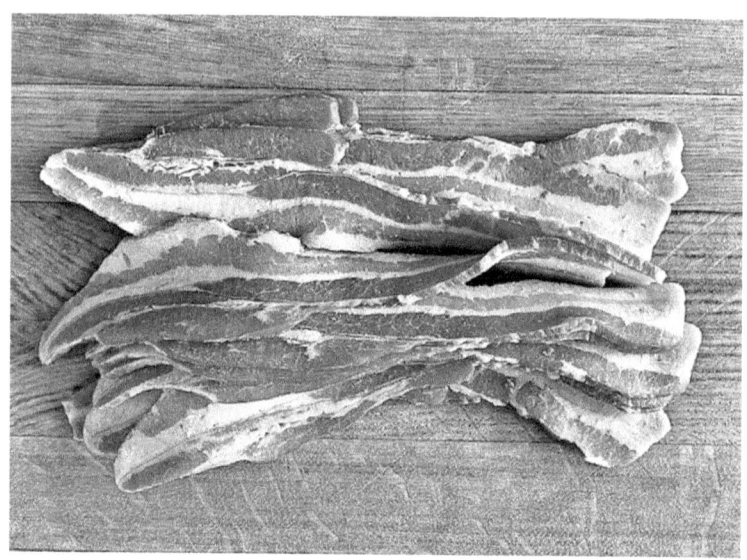

Ingredients:

18 ounces bacon, cut into 1 inch pieces

9 large eggs

8 cups sweet potatoes, chopped into ½ inch cubes

1 ½ cups onion, chopped

6 cups zucchini, chopped into ½ inch cubes

1 large red bell pepper, chopped

Freshly ground black pepper to taste

Salt to taste

2 tablespoons ghee or bacon fat or coconut oil (to be used only if the bacon when cooked does not leave behind fat in the skillet)

Method:

1. Place a large cast iron skillet (that should be able to fit in the oven) over medium low heat. When the skillet is heated, add bacon and cook until crisp. Remove bacon with a slotted spoon and set aside.

2. Increase heat to medium. Add sweet potatoes and do not stir for a few minutes. Pick one sweet potato cube to check if the bottom is golden brown. If so, then stir the sweet potatoes by flipping sides. Cook for a few more minutes until nearly tender.

3. Add onions, zucchini and bell pepper and sauté until the vegetables are slightly tender.

4. Remove from heat. Make 9 cavities (it should fit an egg) in the vegetables in the skillet. Crack an egg into each cavity.

5. Place the skillet in a preheated oven 400° F and bake until the eggs are set (to the way you like it cooked).

6. Remove from the oven and serve

Breakfast Pie

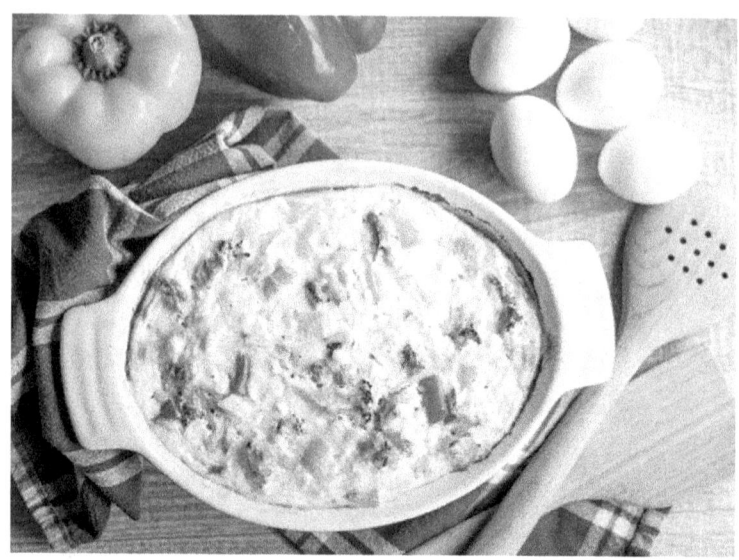

Ingredients:

12 eggs, whisked

1 ½ pounds pork sausages, broken

1 cup sweet potato, shredded

2 onions, chopped

1 cup yellow squash chopped

1 red bell pepper, chopped

1 green bell pepper, chopped

1 tablespoon dried basil

1 tablespoon garlic, minced

Salt to taste

Pepper powder to taste

Cooking spray

Method:

1. Place a skillet over medium heat. Spray cooking spray. Add onions and garlic and sauté for a few minutes until translucent. Add sausages and cook until brown. Break it simultaneously as it cooks.
2. Add squash, the bell peppers, salt and pepper. Remove from heat and transfer into a pie dish. Spread the mixture all over the dish. Press lightly.
3. Pour whisked eggs over it. Sprinkle some salt and pepper.
4. Bake in a preheated oven at 400° F and bake until the eggs are well set. Switch off the oven. Let it remain in the oven for 8-10 minutes
5. Remove from the oven. Slice into wedges and serve.

Paleo Blueberry Muffins

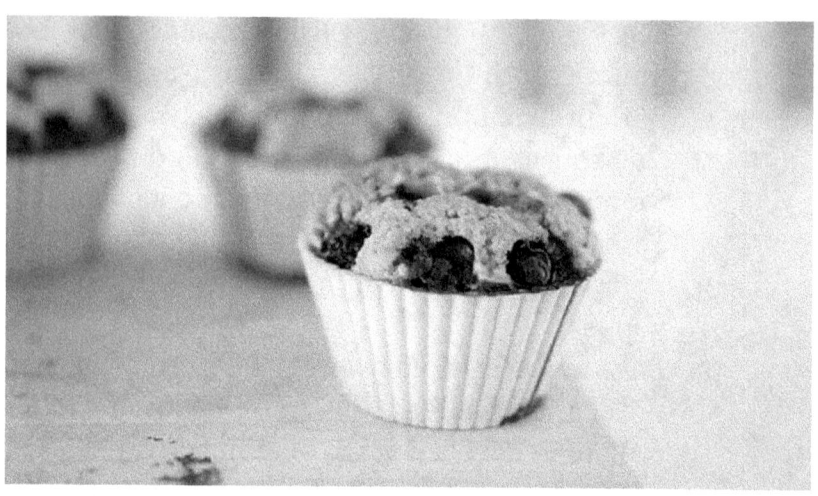

Ingredients:

2 eggs

2 cups blanched almond flour

4 tablespoons raw honey

¼ teaspoon baking soda

¼ cup coconut oil, melted

1 cup full fat coconut milk

½ cup fresh blueberries

1/8 teaspoon salt

2 teaspoons vanilla extract

½ cup nuts of your choice, chopped (optional)

2/3 cup dark chocolate chips (optional)

Method:

1. Mix together in a bowl, almond flour, salt and baking soda.
2. Add honey, coconut milk, eggs and coconut oil to another bowl and whisk well. Pour into the bowl of flour and mix well. It should not be over mixed.
3. Add blueberries and fold gently.
4. Line muffin molds with paper baking cups. Fill batter up to ¾.
5. Bake in a preheated oven at 350° F for about 20 minutes or a toothpick when inserted in the center of the muffin comes out clean.
6. Cool on a wire rack. Cool completely and discard the paper cups and serve.
7. The left over muffins can be packed in an airtight container and stored in the refrigerator.

Savory Casserole

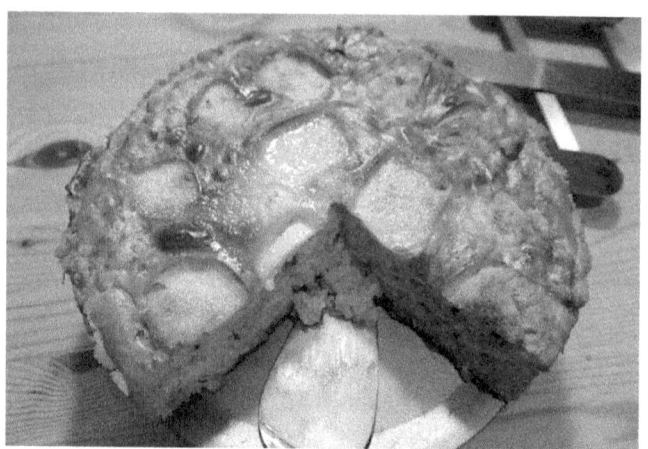

Ingredients:

6 eggs, whisked
1 small sweet potato, shredded
1/2 pound chorizo
1 tablespoon Sriracha sauce
1 small yellow onion, diced
1/2 teaspoon onion powder
1/2 teaspoon garlic powder
1/2 teaspoon pepper powder
1/2 teaspoon salt

Method:

Place a skillet over medium heat. Add chorizo and cook until it crumbles. Remove from heat and set aside.
Add chorizo, and rest of the ingredients to the bowl of whisked eggs. Whisk well.
Pour into a greased baking dish.
Bake in a preheated oven at 300 degree F for 20 minutes or until set. Let it remain in the oven for 10 minutes before serving.

Banana Bread French toast

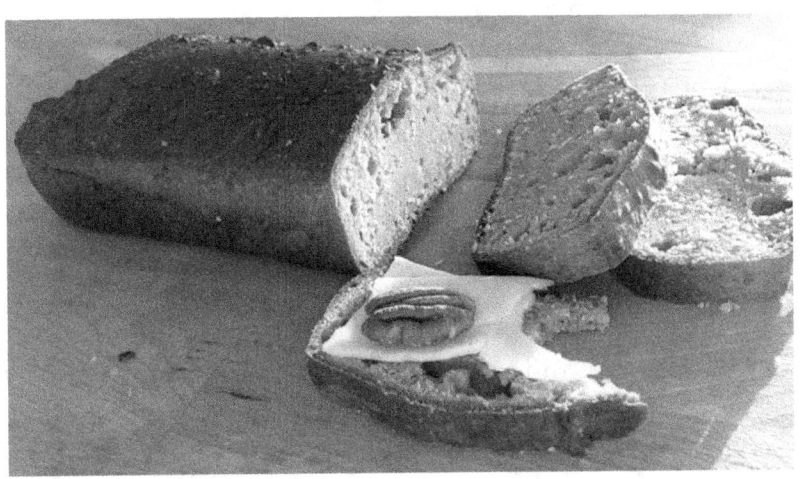

Ingredients:
For the banana bread:

  6 medium very ripe bananas, peeled, chopped

  4 eggs, whisked

  2 cups almond meal or almond flour

  3 cups unsalted cashews, roasted, ground

  2 teaspoons baking powder

  2 teaspoons baking soda

  4 tablespoons walnut oil

  1 teaspoon ground cinnamon

  2 teaspoons vanilla extract

  A pinch salt

For the French toast:

  4 eggs

  2-3 tablespoons coconut oil or as required

  2 teaspoons vanilla extract

  2/3 cup canned coconut milk

  ½ teaspoon cinnamon

<u>To serve:</u>

> Honey or maple syrup
> Ground cinnamon as required

Method:

1. Add ground cashew into the food processor. Add walnut oil and pulse until well combined.
2. Add bananas and pulse until smooth. Transfer into the bowl of eggs. Whisk well.
3. Mix together in a bowl almond meal or flour, baking powder and baking soda. Add this mixture into the bowl of banana mixture. Also add honey, vanilla extract, salt and ground cinnamon. Mix until a smooth batter is formed.
4. Grease a loaf pan with a little coconut oil. Transfer the batter into the loaf pan.
5. Bake in a preheated oven at 375° F for about 30 minutes or until done and the top is brown. Remove from the oven and cool for 10-15 minutes. Cut into slices and set aside.
6. Meanwhile, add all the ingredients of the French toast except coconut oil in a bowl and whisk well.
7. Place a skillet or griddle over medium heat. Add a little coconut oil to it. When the oil is heated, dip the bread slice in the French toast mixture and immediately place on the griddle. Cook until the underside is golden brown. Flip sides and cook the other side too. Remove and place on a serving plate.
8. Sprinkle cinnamon and serve with maple syrup or honey.

Arugula and Leek Frittata

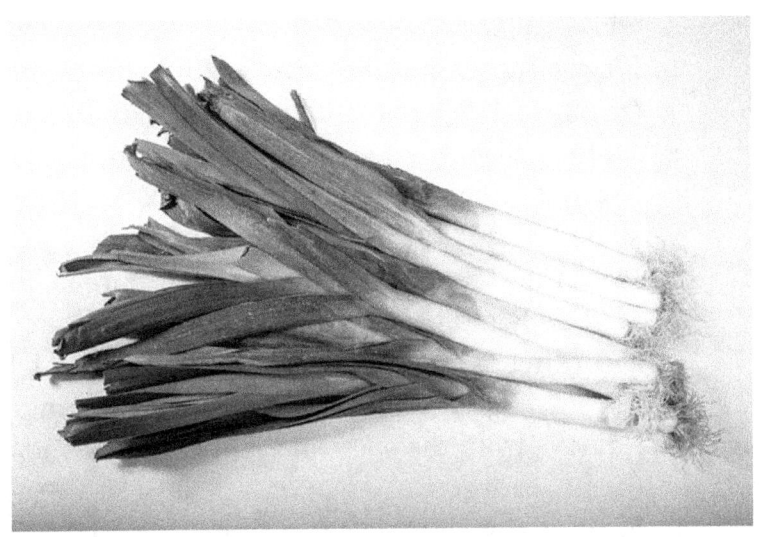

Ingredients:

6 large eggs

2 leeks, sliced

2 cups baby arugula

2 cloves garlic, minced

6 cherry tomatoes, halved

Sea salt to taste

Freshly ground pepper to taste

1 tablespoon coconut oil

1 tablespoon olive oil

¼ cup full fat coconut milk

½ teaspoon balsamic vinegar

Method:

1. Add eggs, coconut milk and salt into a bowl and whisk well.
2. Place a cast iron skillet over medium heat. Add coconut oil. When the oil is heated, add leeks and sauté until soft. Add garlic and sauté until fragrant.
3. Remove from heat. Pour the egg mixture into the skillet. Sprinkle salt and pepper.
4. Place the skillet in an oven. Bake in a preheated oven at 400° F and bake until the eggs are well set according to the way you like it cooked. Switch off the oven. Let it remain in the oven for 4-5 minutes.
5. Remove from the oven and place arugula and tomatoes over it.
6. Whisk together vinegar and olive oil and drizzle over the frittata.
7. Slice into wedges and serve.

Chorizo Mashed Yam

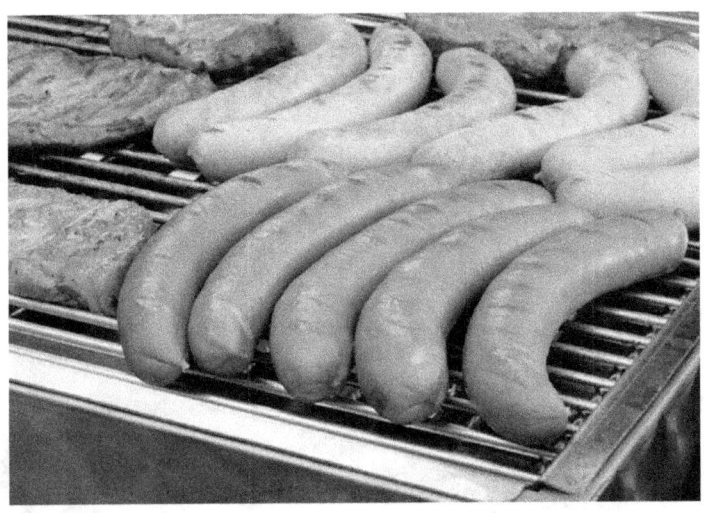

Ingredients:

2 yams, peeled, chopped

1/2 pound Mexican chorizo, discard casings

2 cloves garlic, minced

1 tablespoon butter

1 small onion, chopped

Sea salt to taste

Pepper to taste

2 tablespoons cilantro, chopped

Method:

Melt butter in a saucepan over medium heat. Add onions and sauté until soft. Add garlic and sauté until fragrant.

Add chorizo and cook until light brown.

Place yam in slow cooker. Place chorizo over it.

Cover and set the cooker on High for 3-4 hours.

Discard extra liquid.

Transfer into a bowl, mash and garnish with cilantro.

Tomato Frittata

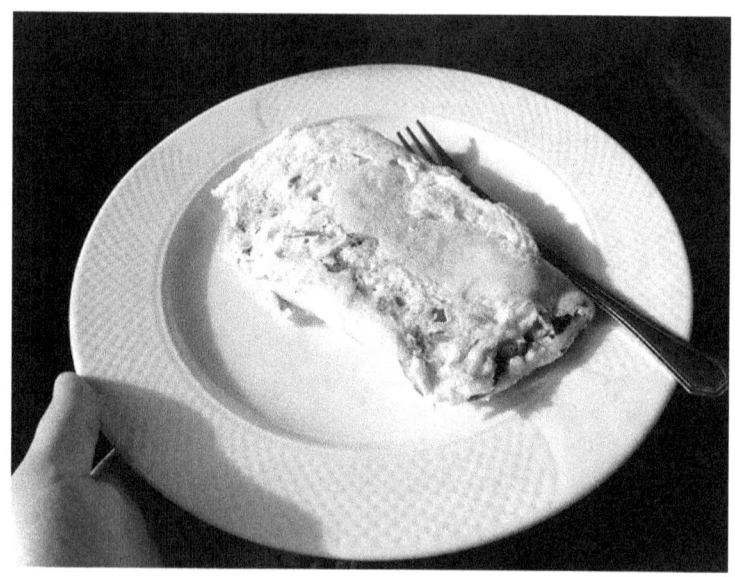

Ingredients:

5 large eggs

3 bacon slices, chopped into small chunks

1 medium sized onions, thinly sliced

2 ounce baby spinach leaves

1 ripe tomato, thinly sliced

1 ½ teaspoon homemade mustard

Fresh basil leaves for garnishing

½ tablespoon olive oil

Sea salt to taste

Pepper powder to taste

Method:

Whisk the eggs well. Add salt and pepper.

Heat olive oil in an ovenproof skillet. When oil is heated, add onions and bacon and sauté until the onions are golden brown.

Add spinach and sauté until the spinach wilts.

Pour the egg mixture over the onion mixture. Cook for about a minute.

Sprinkle tomatoes on top of the egg layer. When the sides are cooked and the middle undercooked, place the skillet in a preheated oven to 350 degree F.

Bake for around 30 minutes or until the top is golden brown.

Garnish with fresh basil leaves. Cut into wedges and serve.

Smoky Pork Carnitas

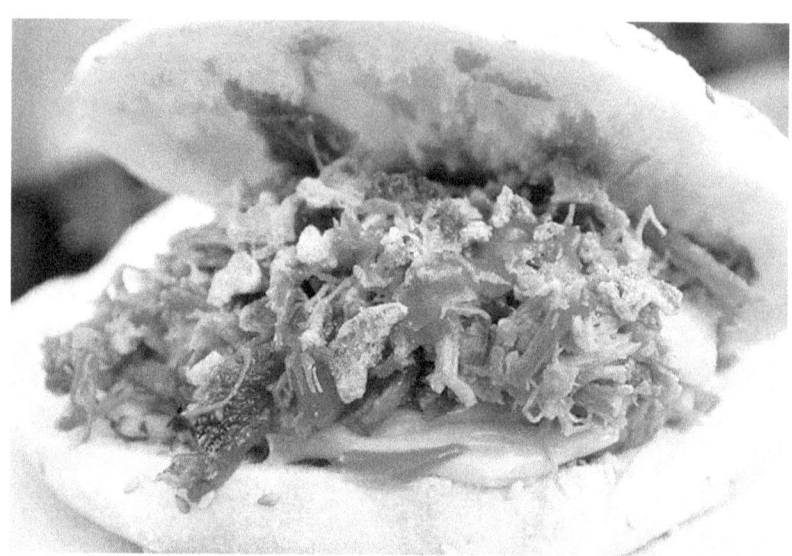

Ingredients:

1 3/4 pounds bone-in-pork shoulder
3/4 cup water
1/2 teaspoon garlic powder
1 teaspoon smoked paprika
1/2 teaspoon dried thyme
1 teaspoon pepper powder
1/2 teaspoon salt

Method:

Mix together all the spices and salt in a bowl. Rub pork with this.
Place in a crockpot. Add water all around.
Cover and cook on Low for 6-8 hours or until tender.
Remove from the crock-pot and place on your cutting board. When cool enough to handle, shred the meat using forks.
Reheat and serve.

Breakfast Meatballs

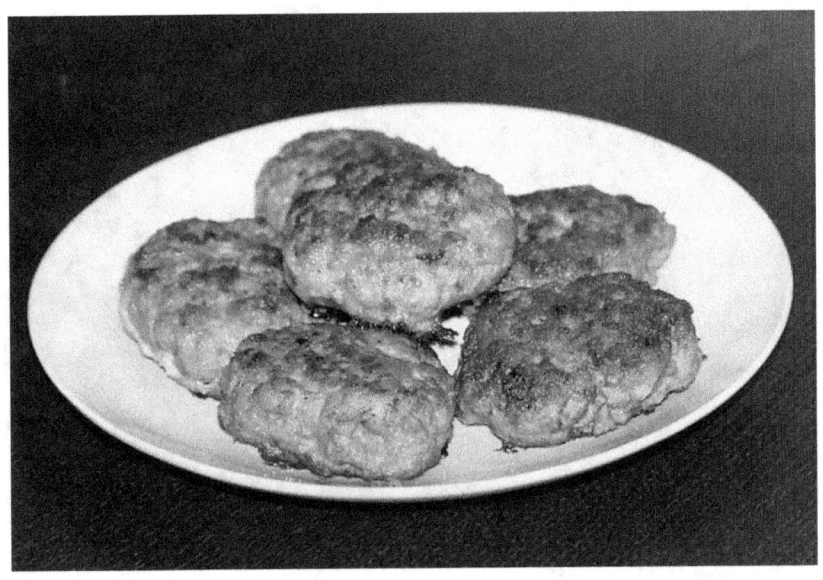

Ingredients

> 1 pound ground beef
>
> 4 eggs
>
> 6 Roma tomatoes
>
> 2 tablespoons nutritional yeast
>
> 4 teaspoons onion powder
>
> 2 red onions, finely chopped
>
> 2 red bell peppers, finely chopped
>
> 2 cloves garlic

Method:

> Place the tomatoes in a preheated grill and set aside
> to keep warm.
>
> Mix rest of the ingredients together.
>
> Shape into small balls and place on a baking sheet.
>
> Bake in a preheated oven at 35 degree F for 25
> minutes or until done.

Chapter 4: Paleo Snacks Recipes

Cajun Cauliflower Mini Dogs

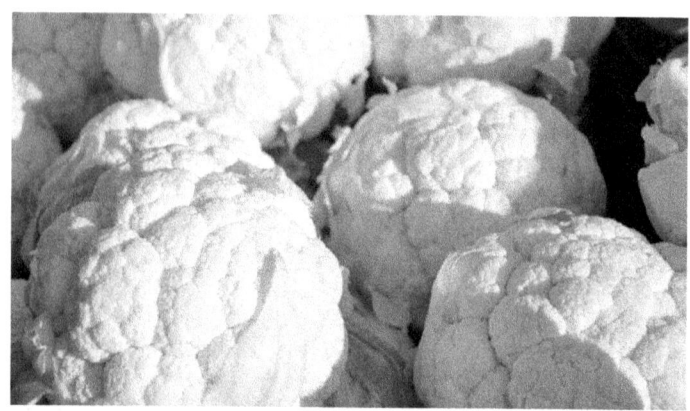

Ingredients:

2 cups cauliflower, grated or ground

24 mini Cajun spiced sausages

4 eggs, beaten

½ cup coconut flour

½ cup non dairy cheese of your choice, grated

1 teaspoon baking soda mixed with 2 teaspoons apple cider vinegar

1 teaspoon ground mustard

2 tablespoons red pepper sauce (optional)

½ teaspoon smoked paprika

¼ teaspoon chili powder

1-2 jalapeños, minced (optional)

3 tablespoons coconut oil or butter, melted

To serve:

Hot sauce

Mustard

Method:

1. Grease a baking sheet with a little oil.
2. Add cauliflower, coconut flour, eggs, paprika, cheese, butter, red pepper sauce, ground mustard, salt, chili powder, jalapeño, baking soda vinegar mixture into a bowl and mix well.
3. Divide the mixture into 24 portions. Take a portion in your hand and flatten it. Place a mini sausage in the middle and cover from all the sides. Place on the baking sheet.
4. Bake in a preheated oven at 400° F for about 20-25 minutes until top is brown and firm.
5. Remove from the oven. Cool for a while. Chop into 2 if desired and serve.
6. Serve with mustard and hot sauce.

Zucchini Fritters

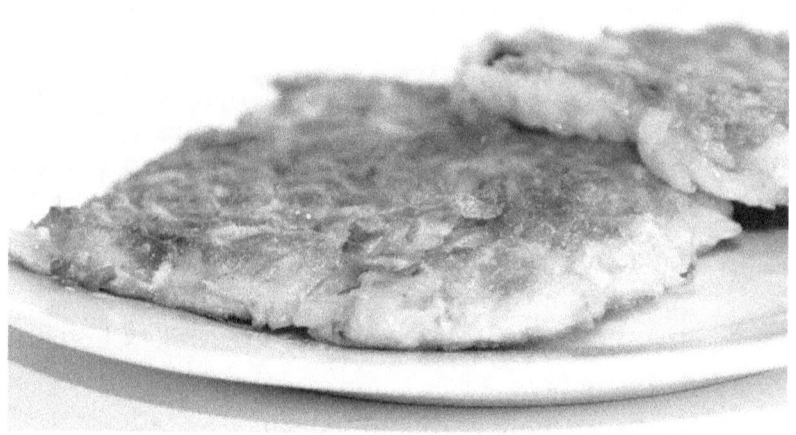

Ingredients:

4 zucchinis, grated

4 tablespoons coconut flour

4 tablespoons coconut oil

2 teaspoons sea salt

Pepper to taste

2 scallions, chopped + extra to garnish

2 teaspoons cayenne pepper

2 eggs

Method:

1. Mix together in a bowl, zucchini and salt and set aside for about 10 minutes.
2. Using your hands, squeeze out the water from the zucchini and place zucchini in a bowl.
3. Add coconut flour, egg, scallions, cayenne and pepper into the bowl. Mix well. Taste and adjust the seasoning if necessary. Divide the mixture into 10-12 portions and form each into patties.
4. Place a skillet over medium high heat. Add about tablespoon of oil. When the oil is heated, place a few of the fritters over it and cook until the bottom side is golden brown. Flip sides and cook the other side too.
5. Remove and place on paper towels.
6. Repeat the above 2 steps with the remaining fritters adding a little oil each time.
7. Serve immediately garnished with scallions. You can also serve with Paleo dips.

Deviled Eggs

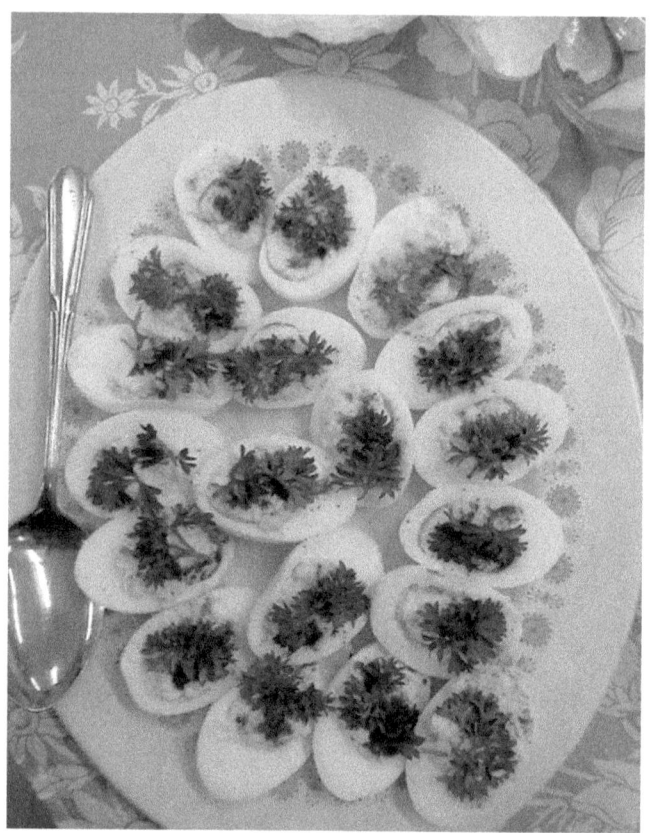

Ingredients:

    6 eggs, hard boiled, peeled, halved

    ¼ cup Paleo mayonnaise

    ½ tablespoon mustard

    ½ tablespoon ground cumin

    3 slices bacon

    ¼ teaspoon paprika

    Sea salt to taste

    Black pepper powder to taste

    Any herbs or seasoning of your choice

Method:

1. Place a nonstick pan over medium heat. Place the bacon slices and cook until crisp. Remove with a slotted spoon.
2. When cool enough to handle, crumble the bacon.
3. Scoop out the yolks from the eggs and keep it aside in a bowl. Set aside the white part.
4. Mash the yolk and add the rest of the ingredients and mix well. Fill the yolk cavities in the white with this filling.
5. Sprinkle paprika and herbs. Place on a serving platter and serve.

Buffalo Chicken Peppers

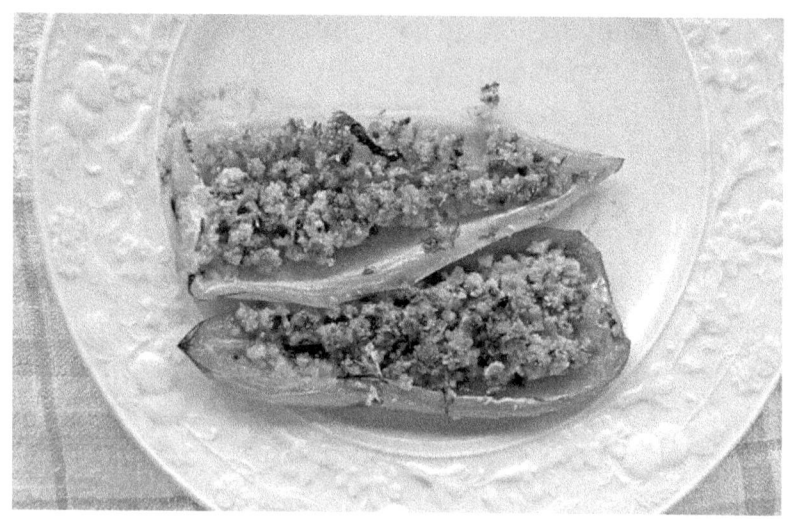

Ingredients:

    2 cups chicken, cooked, shredded

    4 hard boiled eggs, peeled, diced

    12 mini peppers, halved

    1 medium onion, chopped

    2 tablespoons grass fed butter, melted

    Pepper to taste

    2 tablespoons hot sauce

Method:

1. Mix together butter and sauce in a bowl.
2. Add chicken, onion and eggs. Mix well.
3. Stuff the chicken mixture into the peppers. Sprinkle pepper over it.
4. Serve immediately

Chicken Fingers

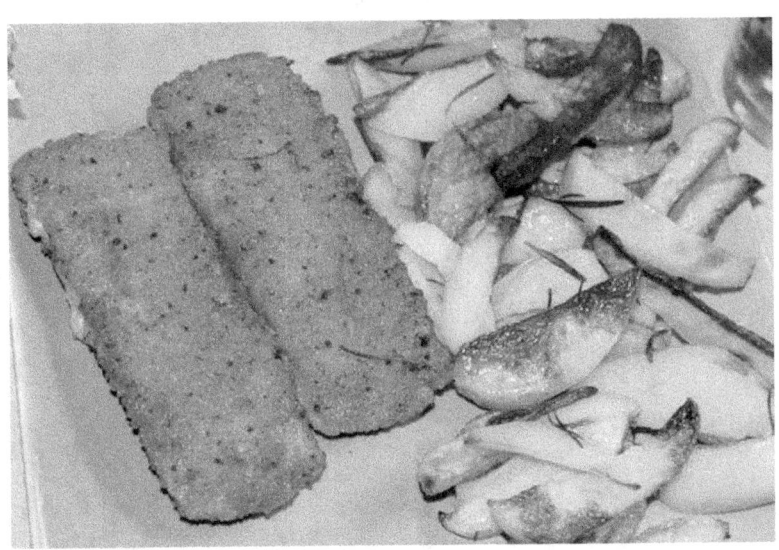

Ingredients:

4 chicken breasts, chop into strips of about 1 inch wide and 3 inches long

4 tablespoons curry powder or to taste

1 1/4 cups coconut flour

3 teaspoons garlic powder

1 teaspoon turmeric powder

3 teaspoons cumin powder

Salt to taste

Method:

1. Mix together the dry ingredients in a bowl.
2. Dredge the chicken pieces in the dry mixture. Shake off the excess mixture and place on a greased baking dish.
3. Bake in a preheated oven at 350 degree F for 20 minutes or until done.

Mashed Sweet Potatoes

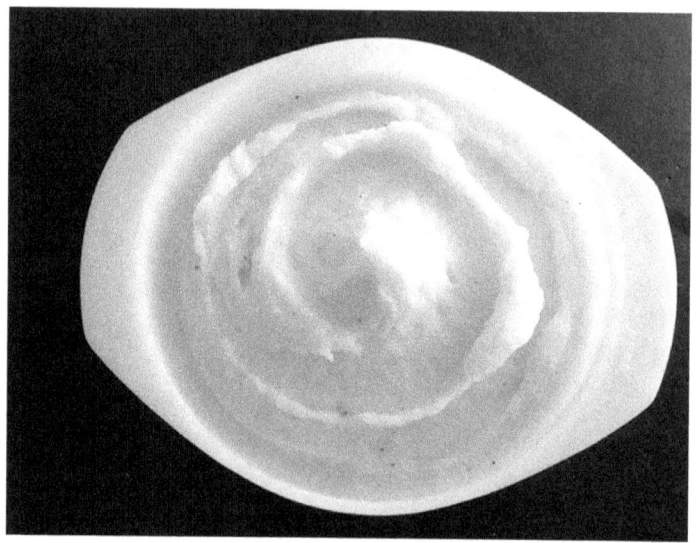

Ingredients:

6 medium whole sweet potatoes (around 4 ½ pounds), rinsed

Freshly ground pepper to taste

Sea salt to taste

1/3 cup ghee or coconut oil or butter

Method:

1. Place the sweet potatoes on a baking sheet. Bake in a preheated oven at 375° F for about 60 minutes or until done.
2. Remove the baking sheet from the oven. When cool enough to handle, peel the skin of the sweet potatoes.
3. Place the sweet potatoes in a serving dish. Mash with a potato masher. Add salt, pepper and melted butter. Stir and serve.

Meat Bagel

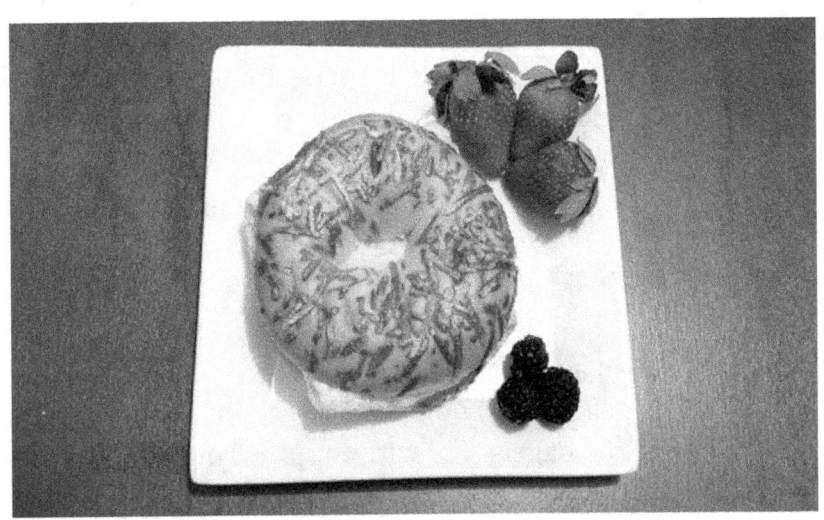

Ingredients:

    1 pound ground pork
    1 medium onion, finely chopped
    1 large egg
    1/3 cup tomato sauce
    ½ tablespoon butter or ghee
    ½ teaspoon paprika
    ¼ teaspoon pepper powder
    ½ teaspoon salt
    Toppings of your choice

Method:

1. Place a skillet over medium heat. Add ghee or butter. When it melts, add onions and sauté until translucent. Remove from heat and cool completely.
2. Transfer into a bowl and add rest of the ingredients and mix well.
3. Divide into 3 or 4 equal portions and shape into a bagel.
4. Place in a baking dish that is lined with parchment paper.
5. Bake in a preheated oven at 400° F for about 40 minutes or until done.
6. Slice the bagels. Fill with toppings of your choice and serve.

Zucchini Pasta / Noodles

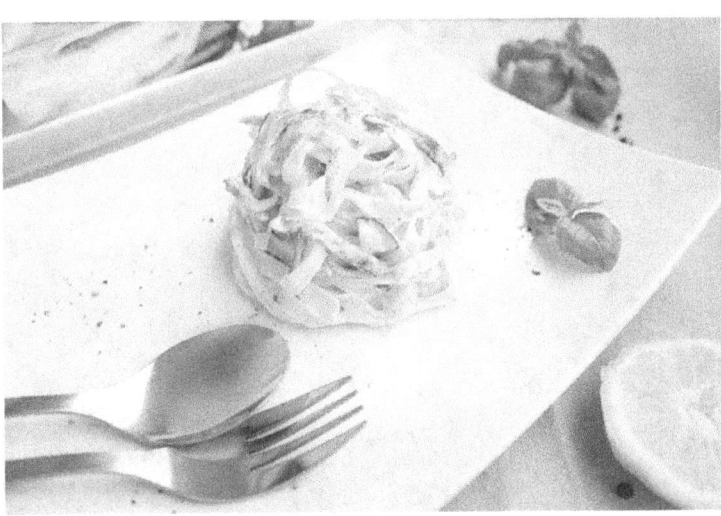

Ingredients:

 4 zucchinis, peeled
 3 tablespoons olive oil
 3-4 tablespoons water
 Salt to taste
 Pepper powder to taste

Method:

1. To make zucchini pasta: Using a vegetable peeler, peel strips of the zucchini lengthwise. Discard the seed part.
2. Place a nonstick pan over medium heat. Add olive oil. When the oil is hot, add the zucchini. Sauté for a couple of minutes. Add water. Cook for a while until the water dries up. Season with salt and pepper. Serve with sauce of your choice.
3. To make noodles: Peel strands of the zucchini with a julienne peeler or make noodles using a spiralizer.
4. Repeat step 2.
5. Serve with pasta sauce of your choice.

Paleo Nachos

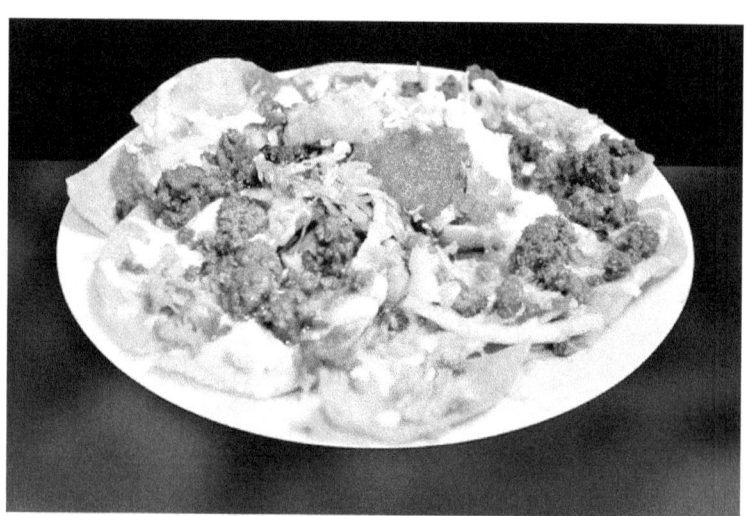

Ingredients:

3/4 pound ground beef

3 cloves garlic, minced

3 teaspoons coconut oil

1 Serrano pepper, chopped

3 tablespoons white onions, minced

1 teaspoon ground cumin

Salt to taste

Pepper powder to taste

Sweet potato chips as required - recipe 177

Guacamole as required

Tomato salsa as required

2 tablespoons fresh cilantro, chopped

3 cups lettuce, shredded

Method:

1. Place a pan with oil over medium heat. Add onion and garlic and sauté until translucent.
2. Add Serrano pepper and beef and cook breaking it simultaneously. Add salt, pepper and cumin and cook until dry.
3. Add most of the cilantro stir and remove from heat.
4. Place chips on a large serving platter.
5. First place lettuce leaves followed by beef mixture followed by salsa and finally guacamole.
6. Garnish with cilantro and serve.

Bacon braised kale

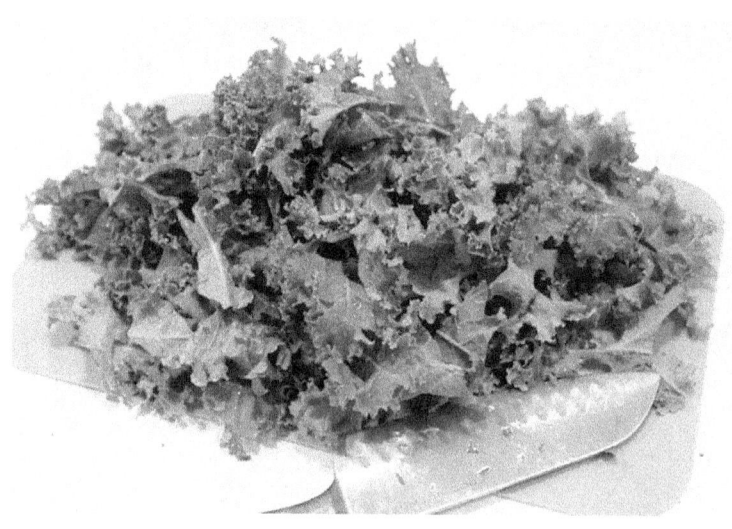

Ingredients:

2 large bunches kale, discard hard stems and ribs
½ to 1 cup broth
6 ounces bacon, chopped into small pieces
2 cloves garlic, crushed
2 tablespoons fresh lemon juice
Salt to taste

Method:

1. Place a skillet over medium high heat. Add bacon and cook until crisp. Remove with a slotted spoon. Retain about 2 tablespoons fat in the skillet and discard the rest.
2. Add kale and about ½ cup broth. Cook until dry. Add a little more broth and cook until kale is tender.
3. Add garlic and lemon juice and sauté for a minute. Serve hot.

Chapter 6: Paleo Main Course Recipes

One Dish Fish and Veggie Bake

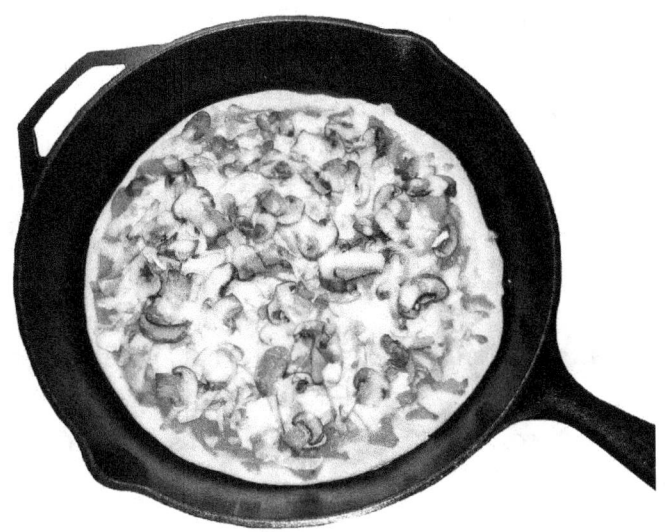

Ingredients:

1 cod fillet or any other fish

2 tablespoons onions, chopped

1 clove garlic, minced

2 tablespoons celery, chopped

1 ½ cups potatoes, diced

1 cup Brussels sprouts, shaved

Sea salt to taste

Freshly ground pepper to taste

¼ teaspoon paprika

2 tablespoons balsamic vinegar

2 tablespoons honey mustard dressing

1 tablespoon fresh lemon juice

2 teaspoons ghee or coconut oil

¼ cup fresh goat's cheese to top

Method:

1. Mix together honey mustard dressing and lemon juice in a bowl. Dip the fillet in it and coat thoroughly. Place the fillet in a baking dish. Set aside for a while.
2. Meanwhile, place a skillet over medium heat. Add ghee. When the ghee melts, add potatoes and cook until slightly tender. Remove from heat. Add onion, garlic, celery and Brussels sprouts and mix well. Add vinegar, paprika, salt and pepper and stir.
3. Place the vegetable mixture over the fillet. Sprinkle goat's cheese over it.
4. Bake in a preheated oven at 450° F for about 15 minutes.
5. Broil for a couple of minutes and serve.

Baked Eggplant with Tomato Thyme Salsa

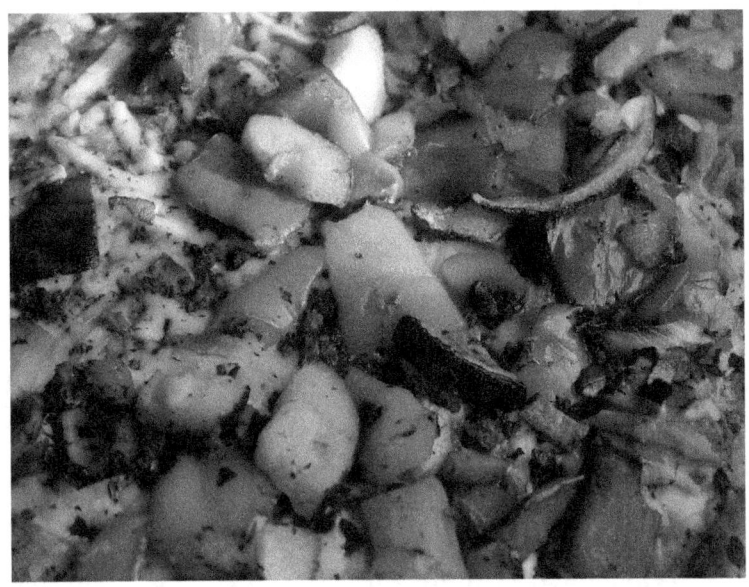

Ingredients:

    2 large eggplants, rinsed, dried

    2 cloves garlic, peeled, minced

    4 medium tomatoes, chopped

    5 tablespoons olive oil + extra to roast and drizzle

    6 sprigs fresh thyme, use only the leaves + extra to garnish

    Freshly cracked pepper to taste

    Sea salt to taste

    Juice of a lemon

Method:

1. Place the whole eggplant on a baking sheet and place in the middle rack of the oven.
2. Bake in a preheated oven at 390° F for about 30 minutes. Remove the eggplant and halve it lengthwise.
3. Lower the temperature to 360° F.
4. Brush oil over it and place the baking sheet back in the oven. Bake for 25-30 minutes or until crisp and brown on top.
5. Remove from the oven and cool. Leave about 5 cm from the edges and bottom and scoop the cooked eggplant and add into a bowl. Add tomatoes, garlic, thyme, salt, pepper, lemon juice and oil and mix until well combined.
6. Fill this mixture into the eggplant cases. Garnish each with thyme. Drizzle some olive oil over it and serve.

Easy Chicken Broccoli Casserole

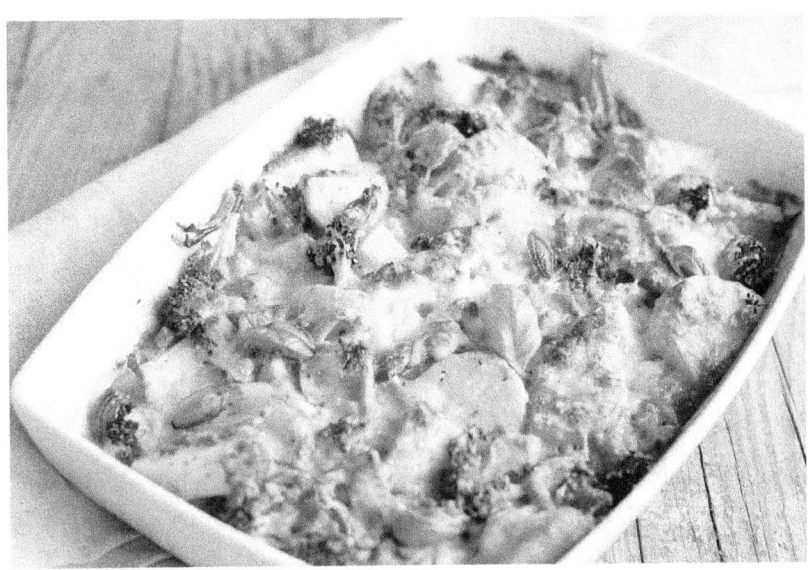

Ingredients:

2 cups broccoli florets, steamed

1 medium onion, chopped

1 ½ cups cooked chicken, shredded

1 egg

4 ounces mushrooms, sliced

1 tablespoon coconut oil, divided

½ cup chicken broth

½ cup full fat coconut milk

¼ teaspoon nutmeg, grated

Salt to taste

Pepper powder to taste

Method:

1. Grease an ovenproof casserole dish with half the coconut oil and set aside.
2. Place a saucepan over medium heat. Add remaining coconut oil. When oil melts, add onions, salt and pepper and cook until brown.
3. Add mushrooms and sauté for another 4-5 minutes. Remove from heat and add broccoli and chicken. Stir and transfer into the casserole dish.
4. Whisk together in a bowl, bone broth, coconut milk, egg, nutmeg, pepper and salt. Pour over the broccoli mixture. Spread it evenly all over.
5. Place the dish in a preheated oven and bake at 350° F for about 35-40 minutes or until set in the center.
6. Remove from the oven. Cool for about 10 minutes and serve.

Paleo Lasagna

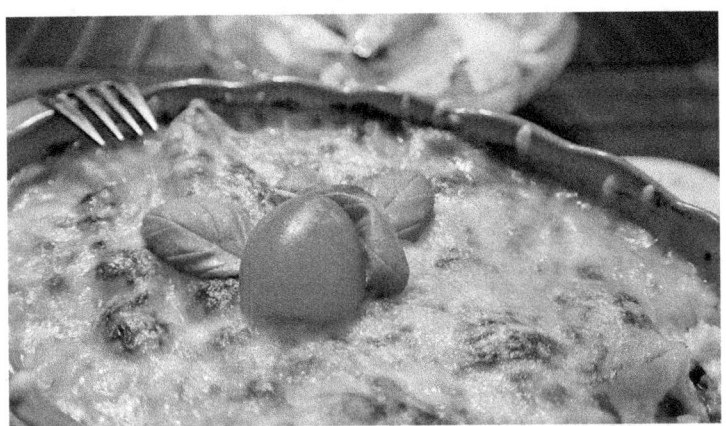

Ingredients:

For the meat sauce:

    ½ pound (30% fat) ground beef

    14 ounces canned crushed tomatoes

    1 teaspoon apple cider vinegar

    2 tablespoons beef stock

    ½ can tomato paste

    1 teaspoon Italian seasoning

    ½ teaspoon onion powder

    ¼ teaspoon garlic powder

    1 bay leaf

    2 drops stevia (optional)

    ¼ teaspoon red crushed pepper

For Lasagna noodles:

    1 small butternut squash

For homemade dairy free cheese:

    4 teaspoons arrowroot starch

    ½ teaspoon lemon juice

    2 tablespoons ghee or tallow

    1 cup almond milk, unsweetened

¼ teaspoon garlic powder

2 eggs, whisked

½ teaspoon onion powder

¾ teaspoon Himalayan rock salt or to taste

½ cup fresh parsley, chopped

Method:

1. Grease a baking dish with coconut oil. Set aside.
2. Place a saucepan over medium heat. Add beef and cook until brown. Add rest of the ingredients of the sauce and stir.
3. Cover and bring to the boil. Lower heat and simmer until thick.
4. Meanwhile make noodles of the butternut squash as follows: Peel the butternut squash and deseed it. Make thin slices of it. Set aside.
5. To make cheese: Mix together all the ingredients of the cheese except ghee, eggs and arrowroot in a bowl.
6. Place a small saucepan over medium heat. Add ghee. When the ghee is melted, add arrowroot. Sauté for 5-7 seconds. Add the mixture in it and stir constantly until smooth and heated thoroughly.
7. Remove from heat and cool for about 15 minutes. Add eggs and whisk until well combined.
8. To assemble the lasagna: Spoon some of the meat sauce at the bottom of the prepared baking dish. Spread a layer of butternut squash noodles. Spread some meat sauce over it. Pour some of the cheese mixture over it. Sprinkle some parsley over it.
9. Repeat the above layer.
10. Bake in a preheated oven at 390° F for about 30 minutes or until the top is set and browned according to the way you desire.

Jordanian Roast Lamb with Tahini Sauce

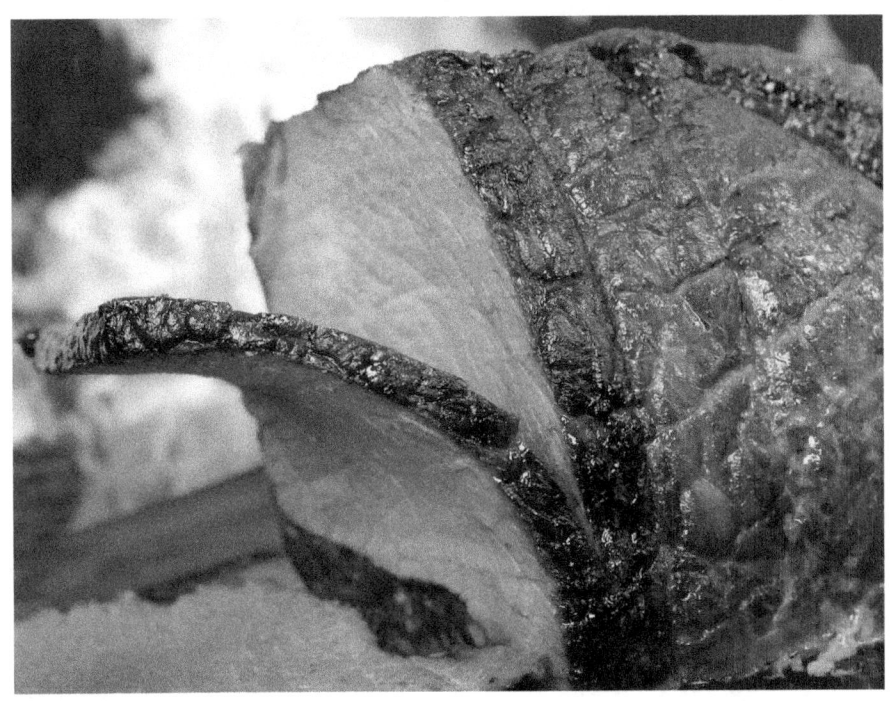

Ingredients:

4 medium cloves garlic, divided

1 1/4 teaspoons salt, divided

1 tablespoon extra-virgin olive oil

3/4 teaspoon ground mace

1/2 teaspoon ground cardamom

1/2 teaspoon paprika

1/2 teaspoon ground cinnamon

1/2 teaspoon ground cumin

1/2 teaspoon cayenne pepper

7 pound boneless leg of lamb, butterflied and trim

1/4 cup lemon juice

1/4 cup tahini sauce

1/4 cup fresh parsley, minced

3 tablespoons coconut yogurt

2 tablespoons water

¼ teaspoon freshly ground pepper

Method:

1. Mince 3 of the garlic cloves. Keep them in a medium bowl with half the salt. Mash mash it to a paste using a spoon.
2. Add oil, cumin, cardamom, mace, paprika, cinnamon, and cayenne. Mix well.
3. Open up the lamb with its cut side up. Spread 3/4 of the above spice mixture over the cut surface.
4. Roll up the lamb and close it. Fasten with threads. Spread the remaining paste on the outside of the roll.
5. Cover loosely with a plastic wrap and refrigerate for 2 hours.
6. Mince the remaining garlic. Mix together the garlic, remaining salt, lemon juice, tahini, parsley, yogurt, water, and pepper. Refrigerate.
7. Meanwhile preheat a gas grill to 400 degree F. You can use a charcoal grill too.
8. If you are using gas grill, then switch off one burner. If you are using charcoal grill, shift the coal to one side.
9. Place the lamb on the unheated side. Cover and roast for 30 minutes. Do not turn it around.
10. After 30 minutes, turn it around, cover and roast for a while. Insert an instant read thermometer in the thickest part of the rolled lamb. It should read 140 degree F. Roast for 20 minutes more.
11. Remove and place on a cutting board. When cool enough to handle, slice it.
12. Serve lamb slices with tahini sauce.

Ground Pork Tacos

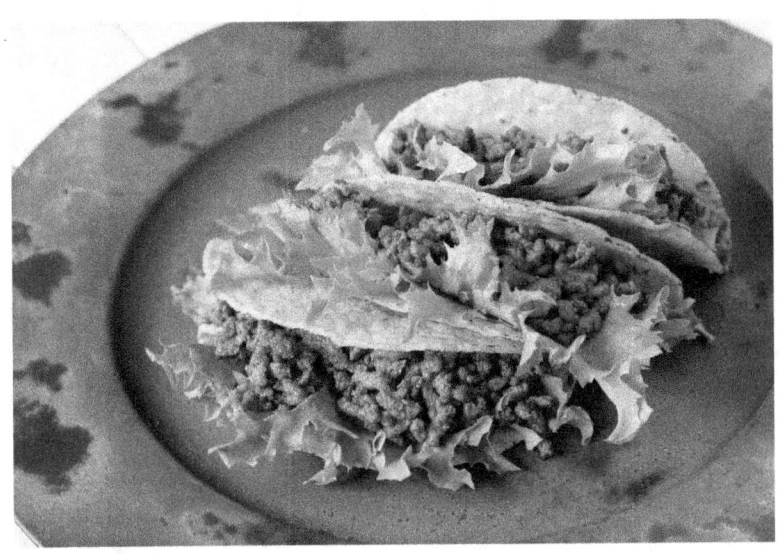

Ingredients:

2 pounds ground pork

1 1/2 teaspoons garlic powder

1 1/2 teaspoons onion powder

1 1/2 teaspoon sea salt

1 teaspoon ground cumin

1/2 teaspoon ground pepper or to taste

1/4 cup salsa

15 large lettuce leaves or more if required

3/4 cup green bell pepper, chopped

3/4 cup red bell pepper, chopped

2 medium onions, chopped

Method:

1. Add pork, garlic powder, onion powder, salt, cumin, and pepper to a skillet. Mix well using your hands.
2. Place the pan over medium heat. Stir constantly and cook until the pork is browned well.
3. Remove the pork with a slotted spoon and place in a bowl. Discard the remaining fat.
4. Add salsa and mix well. Taste and adjust the seasonings if necessary.
5. Lay the lettuce leaves on your working area. Place some pork filling at the center.
6. Sprinkle bell peppers, and onions. Roll and serve.

Roasted Chicken Legs with Vegetables

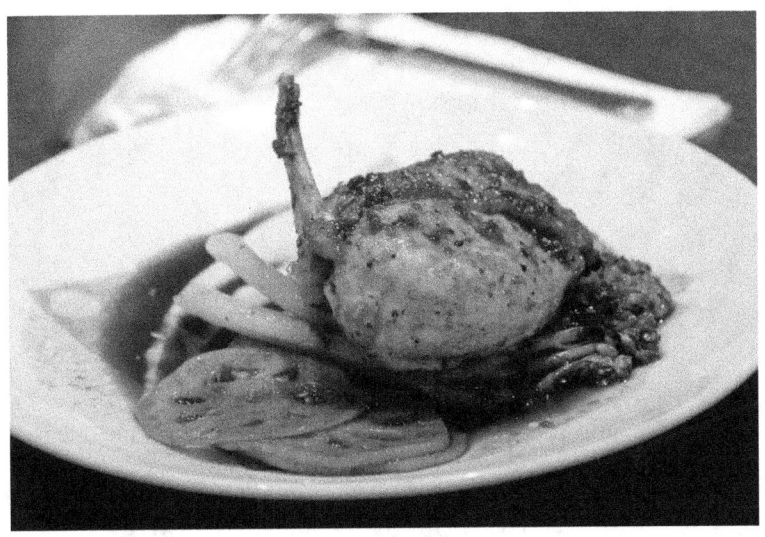

Ingredients:

    8 chicken legs, with skin
    12 cloves garlic, peeled
    8 medium onions, peeled, quartered
    ½ cup olive oil
    ¼ cup lime juice
    ¼ cup fresh parsley
    Sea salt to taste
    Pepper powder to taste

For the vegetables:

    4 cups crimini mushrooms
    4 bell peppers, chopped into 1 ½ inch cubes
    2 cups cherry tomatoes
    4 zucchini, sliced into 1 centimeter thick slices
    6 cloves garlic, minced
    2 red onions, quartered

½ cup olive oil

¼ cup lime juice

1 teaspoon dried basil

1 teaspoon dried oregano

Sea salt to taste

Pepper powder to taste

Skewers as required

Method:

1. Place the chicken legs in a large baking dish. Add onions, garlic, olive oil, lemon juice, salt, pepper and parsley. Mix well.
2. Place the baking dish in an oven. Roast in a preheated oven at 400° F for about 45 minutes. Remove from the oven and keep warm.
3. For the vegetables: In a bowl mix together olive oil, garlic, lime juice, oregano, basil, salt and pepper.
4. Fix the mushrooms, bell peppers, onions, zucchini and tomatoes on to skewers.
5. Place the skewers on a baking sheet. Apply the olive oil mixture over the vegetables with a brush.
6. Roast in the oven for 10 minutes or until the crunchiness of the vegetables you desire is achieved.
7. Serve the chicken with vegetables.

Pan grilled Lamb Chops and Cardoons

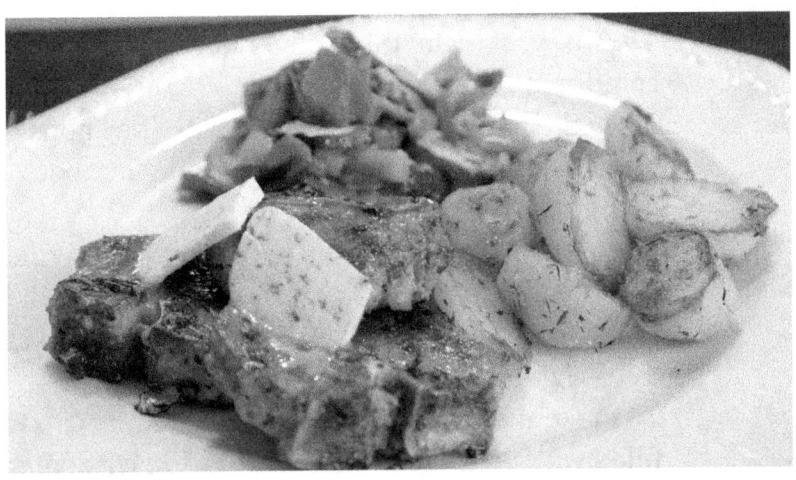

Ingredients:

> 5 lamb shoulder chops
> 5 cloves garlic
> 5 sprigs fresh rosemary
> 5 tablespoons olive oil
> Celtic sea salt to taste

For cardoons:

> 4 bunch cardoons, peel the outer hard skin, cut into
> 4 inch long pieces
> Celtic sea salt to taste

Method:

1. To make the lamb chops: Blend together garlic, rosemary, salt and oil in a blender until well combined

2. Place the lamb chops in a bowl. Rub the chops with the oil mixture. Cover and keep aside for about ½ an hour.

3. Place a cast iron skillet over medium heat. When the skillet is hot, add lamb chops and cook on both the sides until done. Remove the lamb pieces and keep aside. Let the juices remain in the skillet.

4. To make the cardoons: Place a large saucepan with filled with water to boil. Add salt. Add cardoons and cook until tender. Drain and keep aside.

5. Place the skillet back on heat. Add the cooked cardoons. Heat thoroughly.

6. Serve the lamb chops topped with cardoons.

Paleo Spaghetti Squash Hawaiian Pizza Pie

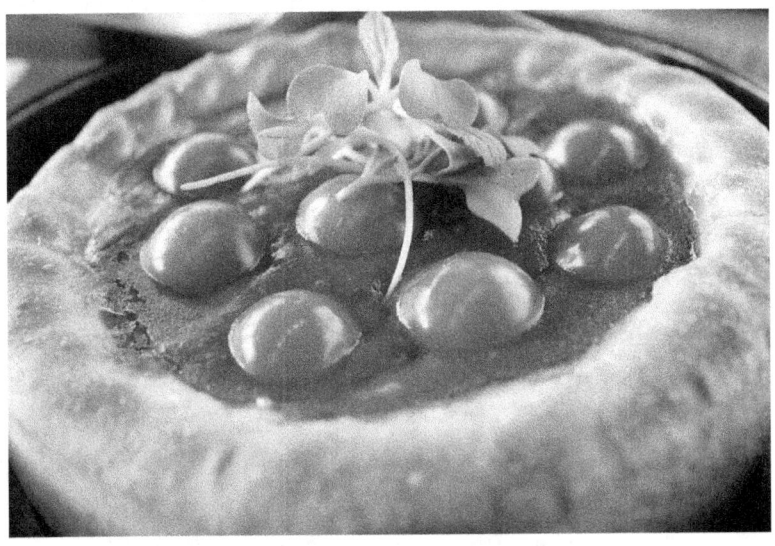

Ingredients:

½ ham steak, diced

1 small spaghetti squash, halved

1 cup pineapple, chopped

1 small onion, chopped

1 large egg, whisked

½ cup pizza or pasta sauce

2 tablespoons fresh basil, chopped

Salt to taste

Pepper powder to taste

1 tablespoon coconut oil

Cooking spray

Method:

1. Place the spaghetti squash in a microwave safe bowl with its cut part touching the bottom of the bowl. Pour enough water (2 inches from the bottom of the bowl).
2. Place in the microwave and microwave on high for 5-8 minutes or until squash is soft.
3. Remove the bowl and discard the water. Set aside to cool. When cool enough to handle, discard the seeds and pull the flesh of the squash with a fork.
4. Meanwhile, place a pan over medium heat. Add oil. When the oil is heated, add ham and onion and sauté until onions are soft and the ham is brown. Remove from heat. Add pizza sauce and mix well. Add pineapple and squash and mix again
5. Spray a small casserole dish with cooking spray. Add squash - ham mixture into the casserole dish and spread it all over the dish. Press lightly.
6. Pour egg over it. Sprinkle salt, pepper and basil.
7. Place the dish in a preheated oven and bake at 400° F for about 50-60 minutes.
8. Slice and serve.

Irish Style Shepherd's Pie

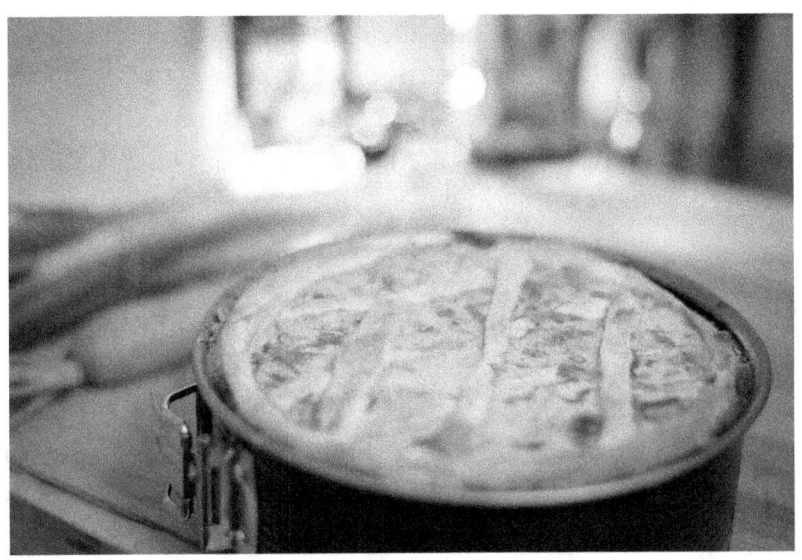

Ingredients:

¾ pound ground beef

1 large carrot, peeled chopped

1 pound russet potatoes or sweet potatoes, peeled, chopped

1 stalk celery, diced

1 small onion, chopped

1 large clove garlic, minced

2 tablespoons dry red wine (optional)

1 fresh bay leaf

1 fresh thyme sprigs

1 tablespoons tomato paste

1 cup beef stock

2 tablespoon ghee

2 tablespoons fresh parsley, chopped

Sea salt to taste

Freshly ground pepper to taste

Method:

1. Place a large pot filled with water. Add either potatoes or sweet potatoes to it and bring to the boil.

2. Lower the heat slightly and simmer until the potatoes are cooked. Remove from heat. Drain the water and add it back into the pot. Add ghee, salt and pepper and mash. Set aside.

3. Place a skillet over medium heat. Add ghee. When the ghee melts, add beef and sauté until brown. Add onions, garlic, celery and carrots and sauté for 2-3 minutes.

4. Add rest of the ingredient except parsley and stir. Cover and cook until the vegetables are soft. Discard the thyme sprig and bay leaf.

5. Transfer the mixture into a baking dish. Spread the mashed potatoes or mashed sweet potatoes over it. Garnish with parsley.

6. Place the dish in a preheated oven and bake at 375° F for about 25-30 minutes.

7. Slice and serve.

Sichuan Style Shrimp

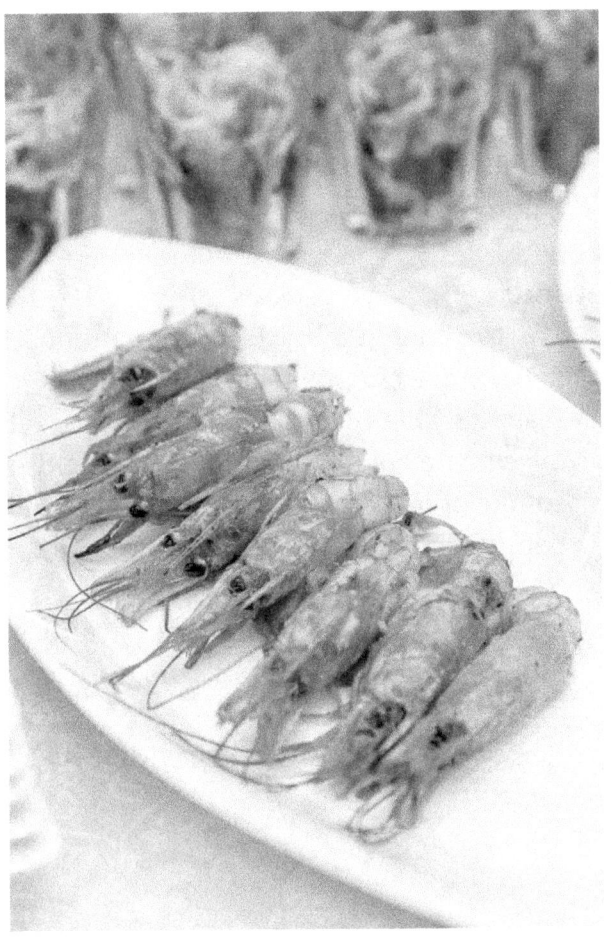

Ingredients:

    30-40 medium shrimp, peeled, deveined
    1 bell pepper, minced
    4 inches fresh ginger, peeled, minced
    1 onion, minced
    2 cloves garlic, minced
    8-9 dry red chilies
    4 tablespoons coconut oil

¼ cup water

½ cup coconut aminos

2 teaspoons apple cider vinegar

2 teaspoons raw honey

2 tablespoons lime juice

A handful of fresh cilantro to garnish

Salt to taste

Method:

1. Mix together in a bowl, coconut aminos, honey, lime juice, apple cider vinegar and water.
2. Place a skillet over medium heat. Add oil. When the oil is heated, add ginger and garlic and sauté for a couple of minutes until fragrant. Add onions, bell pepper and red chilies and sauté until onions are translucent.
3. Add shrimp and cook until the shrimp is cooked and pink in color. Add the sauce mixture and cook until thick.
4. Remove from heat. Garnish with fresh cilantro and serve.

Sesame – Ginger Chicken

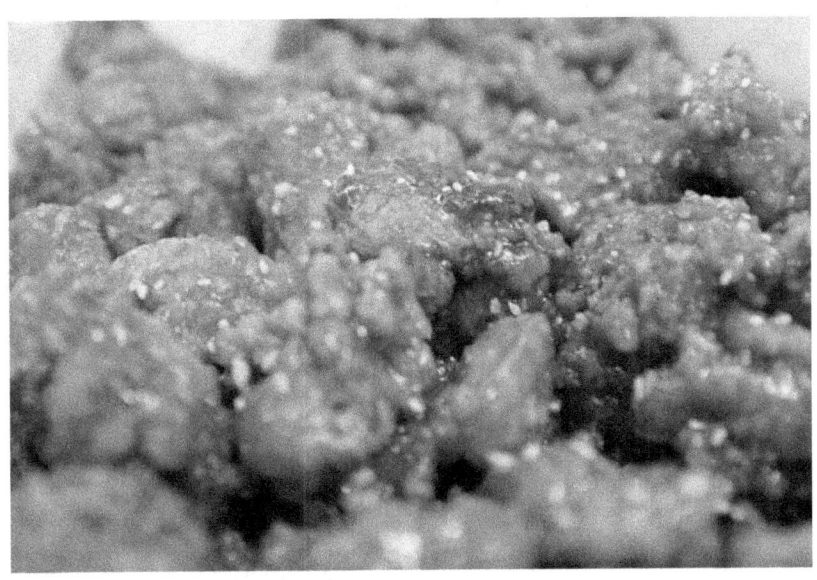

Ingredients:

½ tablespoon sesame oil

4 bone in chicken thighs, skinned

1 tablespoon vegetable oil

2 tablespoons low tamari sauce

1 tablespoon coconut sugar

1 tablespoon fresh orange juice

2 ½ teaspoons hoisin sauce

1 tablespoon ginger, minced

2 cloves garlic

½ tablespoon arrowroot

½ tablespoon water

1 teaspoon sesame seeds toasted

1 tablespoon green onion, sliced

Cooking spray

Method:
1. Place a nonstick skillet over medium heat. Add oil and heat. Add chicken and cook on both sides until golden brown.
2. Spray the slow cooker with oil. Place the browned chicken in the cooker.
3. Mix together tamari sauce, coconut sugar, orange juice, hoisin sauce, ginger, and garlic. Pour this over the chicken. Cover.
4. Set the cooker on Low for 2 ½ to 3 hours. Transfer the chicken on to a platter and keep warm.
5. Strain the remaining liquid in the cooker and place in a pan (it should measure at least ½ to ¾ cup otherwise add water). Discard the solids.
6. Heat the saucepan over medium heat and bring to a boil. Mix together arrowroot and water in a small bowl. Add this to the saucepan. Stir constantly until thickened. Bring back to a boil.
7. Pour sauce over the chicken.
8. Sprinkle sesame seeds and green onions.

Chicken Adobo

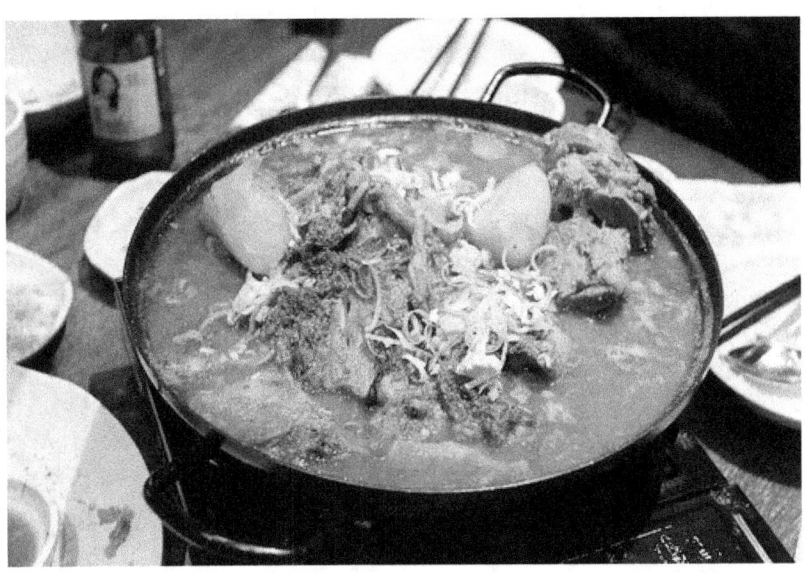

Ingredients:

1 pound chicken thighs, skinless, boneless

2 tablespoons coconut oil

1 red onion, chopped

1/4 cup chicken broth

2 tablespoons coconut aminos or tamari

2 tablespoons apple cider vinegar

Salt to taste

Pepper powder to taste

Salad greens of your choice to serve

Method:

1. Place a skillet with oil over medium heat.
2. When the oil is heated, add the chicken. Cook on both the sides until brown.
3. Remove the chicken with a slotted spoon and keep aside.
4. Add onions to the same skillet. Sauté the onions until pink. Add garlic and sauté for a few more seconds until fragrant.
5. Add broth, tamari and vinegar. Mix well and simmer for a few minutes.
6. Add the chicken and mix well. Reduce heat, cover and simmer for 5-6 minutes.
7. Flip the chicken and cook the other side too for 5-6 minutes.
8. Sprinkle salt and pepper. Serve with greens.

Bottle gourd with Tomatoes

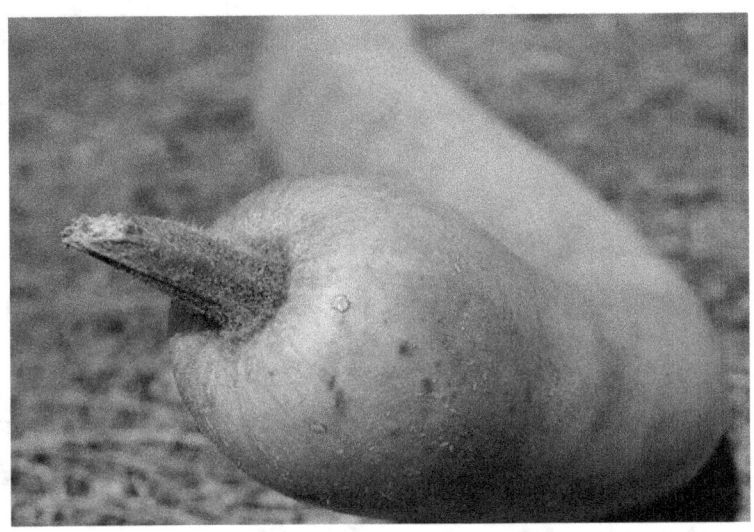

Ingredients:

> 1 medium bottle gourd, peeled, chopped
> 2 large tomatoes
> 1 teaspoon cumin seeds
> 1 tablespoon ghee
> 1/4 teaspoon asafetida
> 1/2 teaspoon chili powder
> 1/2 teaspoon salt or to taste

Method:

1. Place a skillet over medium heat. Add ghee. When ghee is heated, add cumin seeds. It will begin to crackle.
2. Add asafetida. Sauté for 5-6 seconds and add tomatoes. Sauté for a couple of minutes.
3. Add bottle gourd and sauté for a couple of minutes. Add chili powder and salt and stir. Add a cup of water.
4. Stir, cover and cook until bottle gourd is tender. Serve over cauliflower rice

Salisbury Steak with Mushroom Gravy

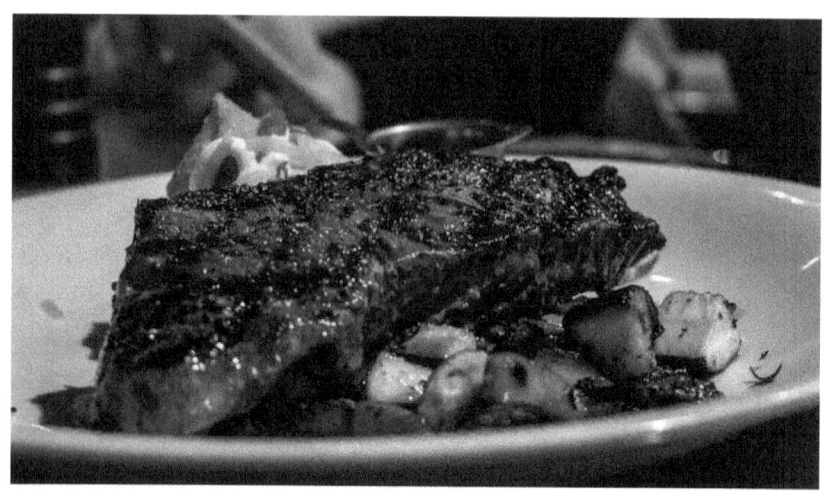

Ingredients:

For steak:

      3/4 pound ground turkey

      2 teaspoons coconut oil

      1 clove garlic, minced

      1 small onion, chopped

      1/2 teaspoon paprika

      1/2 teaspoon fennel seeds

      1/2 teaspoon rosemary

      1/2 teaspoon salt

      1/2 teaspoon pepper

For gravy:

      1 cup mushrooms, chopped

      1/4 cup light coconut milk

      2 teaspoons coconut flour or arrowroot mixed with 2 tablespoons water

      1 cup beef broth

      Salt to taste

      Pepper to taste

Method:

1. Mix together in a bowl, ground turkey, onion, garlic, salt, and spices. Divide and form into patties.
2. Place a nonstick pan over medium heat. Add oil. When oil is heated, add patties and cook until the underside is brown. Flip sides and cook the other side too.
3. Remove from the pan and keep warm.
4. Add mushrooms to the same pan. Sauté until mushrooms are softened.
5. Add broth, coconut milk, salt, and pepper and bring to a boil.
6. Add arrowroot mixture stirring constantly until thickened.
7. Place the steaks on a serving platter. Pour sauce over it and serve.

Zucchini Pasta Bolognese

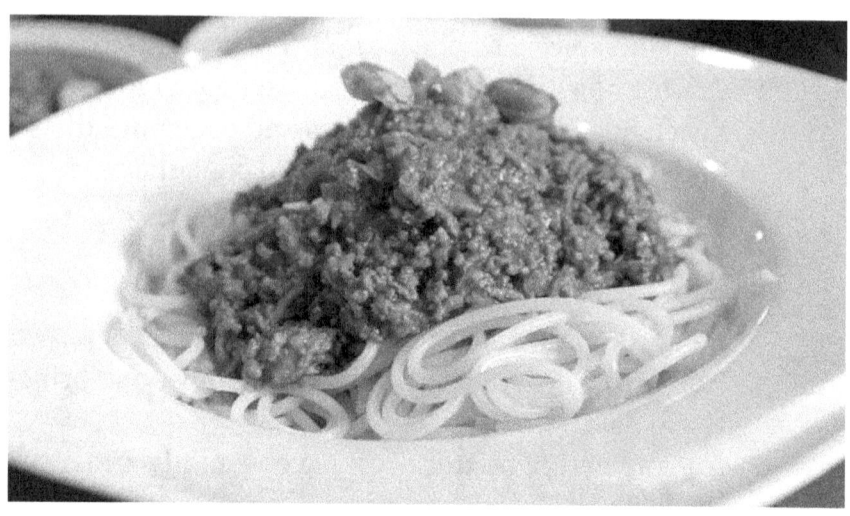

Ingredients:

5 whole zucchinis

1 can tomato paste

2 cans (14.5 ounces each) diced tomatoes

2 large yellow onions, grated

4 cloves garlic, crushed

2 pounds ground lamb

2 cups beef broth or chicken broth

1/3 cup coconut milk

2 cups red wine

2 tablespoons coconut aminos or tamari

2 tablespoons dried oregano

1/2 cup fresh basil leaves, chopped

Salt to taste

Pepper powder to taste

2 tablespoons olive oil or coconut oil

Method:

1. Make noodles of zucchinis by using a spiralizer or a julienne peeler and keep it aside.
2. Place a large saucepan over medium heat. Add oil. When oil is heated, add grated onions.
3. Sauté for a while. Add salt, pepper, and dried oregano and sauté for a couple of minutes.
4. Add garlic and sauté for a couple of minutes until fragrant. Add ground lamb and stir constantly. When beef is light brown, push the lamb all around the pan making space at the center.
5. Add tomato paste in the center and fry for a couple of minutes and slowly mix it in the beef. Add red wine and mix well. Let it cook for a while until the wine almost dries up.
6. Add tomatoes, stock and tamari. Add coconut milk, stir and simmer for 5 minutes.
7. Add basil, stir and simmer for 2-3 minutes.
8. Place the zucchini noodles over individual serving plates. Pour sauce over the noodles and serve

Carrots and Rutabaga Mash

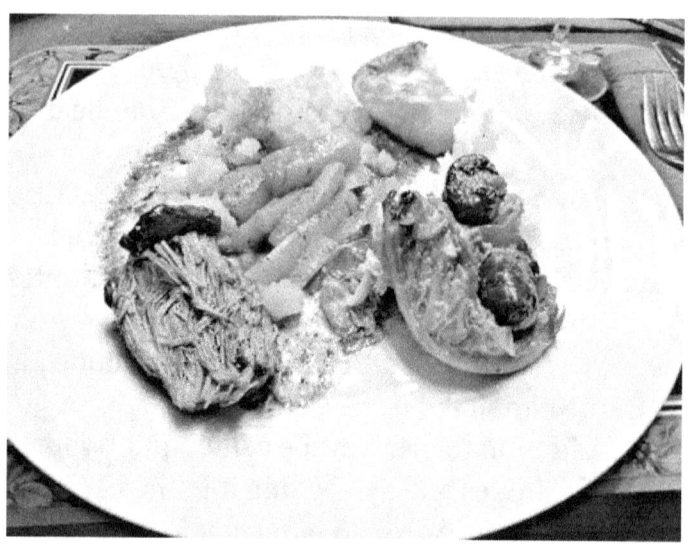

Ingredients:

    2 pounds rutabaga, peeled, chopped
    2 pounds carrots, peeled, chopped
    1/2 cup ghee
    2 tablespoons fresh parsley, minced
    Sea salt to taste
    Pepper powder to taste

Method:

1. Place a large saucepan or pot over medium heat. Add carrots and rutabaga. Cover the saucepan with water and bring to a boil.
2. Lower heat, cover and simmer until the vegetables are very soft. Drain the water and place carrots and rutabaga in a bowl.
3. Mash the cooked carrots and rutabaga with a potato masher. Add ghee, salt and pepper and mix well.
4. Sprinkle fresh parsley and serve.

Slow-Cooker Pepper Steak

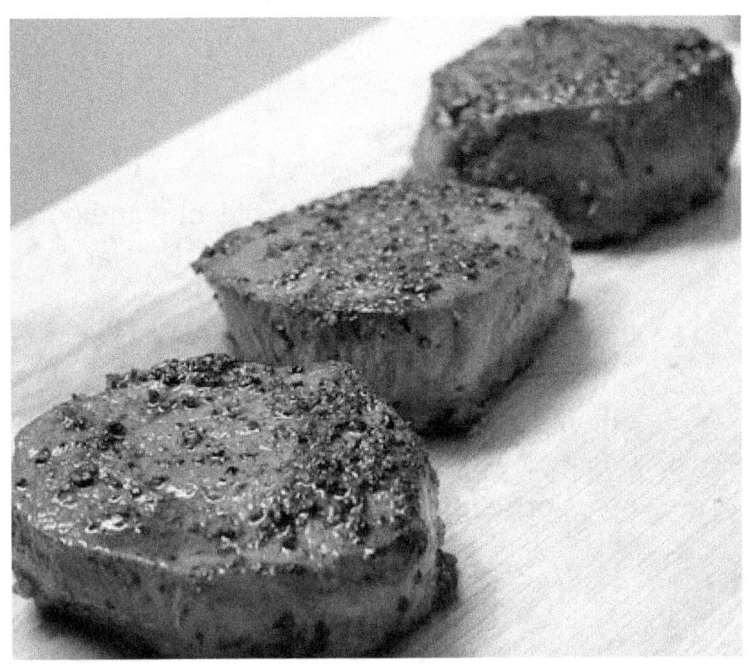

Ingredients:

1 pound beef sirloin, cut into 2 inch strips

1 teaspoon garlic powder or to taste

1 ½ tablespoons coconut oil

½ cube beef bouillon

2 tablespoons hot water

½ tablespoon arrowroot

¼ cup chopped onion

1 large green bell peppers, roughly chopped

½ of a 14.5 ounce can stewed tomatoes, with liquid

1 ½ tablespoons tamari

½ teaspoon coconut sugar

½ teaspoon salt

Method:
1. Sprinkle garlic powder over beef sirloin.
2. Over medium heat place a skillet. Add oil, heat. Add the beef sirloin.
3. Sauté till you brown it.
4. Transfer into a slow cooker.
5. Meanwhile in a bowl, add hot water and bouillon cube. When it is completely dissolved, add arrowroot. Mix well.
6. Pour this mixture into the slow cooker.
7. Add onion, stewed tomatoes, bell pepper, soy sauce salt and sugar.
8. Cover. Set the cooker on High and cook for 4 to 5 hours or set on Low and cook for 7 to 8 hours.

Ratatouille (Vegan)

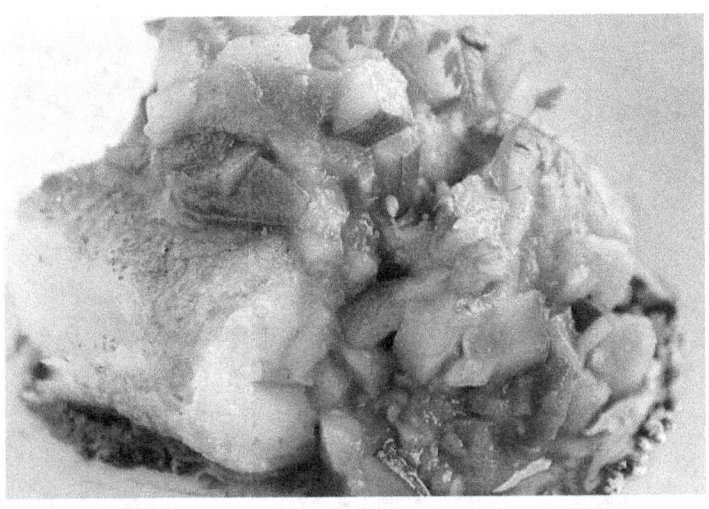

Ingredients:
1 yellow bell pepper, chopped into 2 cm cubes
1 red bell pepper, chopped into 2 cm cubes
1 tomato, chopped into 2 cm cubes
1 courgette, chopped into 2 cm cubes
1 zucchini, chopped into 2 cm cubes
1 large onion, chopped into 2 cm cubes
1 aubergine, chopped into 2 cm cubes
1/2 tablespoon olive oil
1 clove garlic, crushed
1 teaspoon dried Provencal herbs
Freshly ground black pepper
Salt to taste

Method:
1. Mix together courgette, zucchini, aubergine, bell peppers, tomatoes, and onions in a baking dish.
2. Add garlic, oil, herbs, salt and pepper.
3. Place the baking dish in a preheated oven and bake at 350 degree F for about 30 minutes or until done.

Sausage and Cauliflower Bake

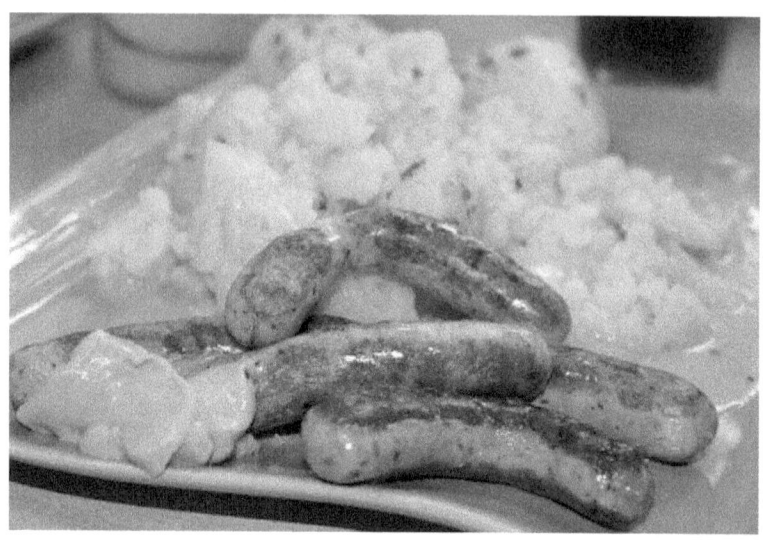

Ingredients

    1 large cauliflower, chopped into florets, steamed

    8 pork sausages

    10 tablespoons coconut cream

    8 slices nondairy cheese

    1 teaspoon salt or to taste

    Pepper powder to taste

Method

1. Mash cauliflower with a potato masher.
2. Add coconut cream, salt and pepper.
3. Place a nonstick skillet over medium heat. Add sausages and cook until done.
4. When cool enough to handle, slice the sausages and add to cauliflower mixture and mix well.
5. Now layer as follows:
6. Add half the cauliflower mixture to a greased baking dish.
7. Lay half the cheese slices.
8. Spread the remaining mixture over the cheese slices.
9. Lay the remaining cheese slices over the cauliflower layer.
10. Place the baking dish in a preheated oven and bake at 350 degree F for around 30 minutes.

Chapter 7: Paleo Dessert Recipes

Apple, Almond & Blackberry Cake

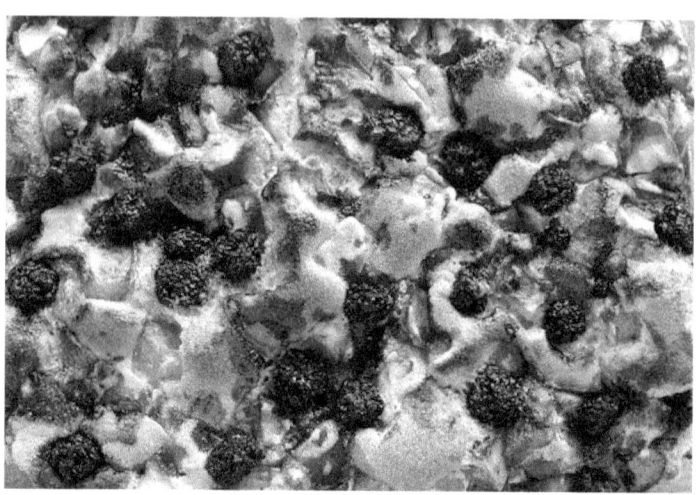

Ingredients:
<u>For the filling:</u>

> 6 apples, peeled, cored, chopped into chunks
>
> 2 tablespoons coconut sugar
>
> 1 cup blackberries
>
> 5-6 tablespoons butter or coconut oil
>
> ¼ teaspoon ground cloves or allspice
>
> 1 teaspoon ground cinnamon
>
> ¼ teaspoon ground ginger
>
> ½ teaspoon ground cardamom

<u>For the batter:</u>

> 1 ½ cups almonds, ground
>
> 2 eggs, whisked or 2 tablespoons chia seeds mixed with 4 tablespoons water and set aside for 10-15 minutes
>
> 4 tablespoons coconut sugar

A pinch salt

1 teaspoon baking powder

1/3 cup coconut milk

2 tablespoons coconut oil or butter

1 teaspoon ground vanilla

Method:

1. To make the filling: Place an ovenproof skillet over high heat. Add butter, apples, cloves or allspice, cinnamon, ginger, cardamom and sugar.
2. Cook until apples are tender and the mixture is caramelized. Remove from heat and set aside.
3. Meanwhile make the batter as follows: Mix together in a bowl, almond flour, ground vanilla, salt, baking powder and sugar. Add egg or chia mixture, coconut milk and coconut oil and stir well.
4. Add blackberries into the skillet of apples and mix well. Pour the batter over it.
5. Bake in a preheated oven at 4000° F for about 15-20 minutes. The top of the cake should be golden brown when the cake is ready.
6. Remove from the oven.
7. Slice and serve warm with some coconut cream or coconut milk.

Pumpkin Pie Ice cream

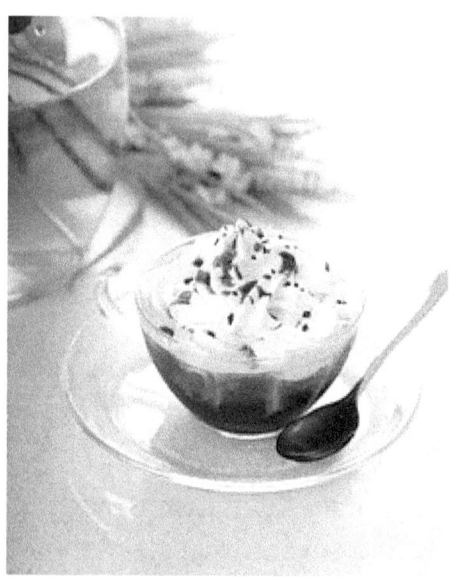

Ingredients:

1 cup pumpkin puree

2 teaspoon pumpkin pie spice

2 cups unsweetened almond milk

2 teaspoons vanilla extract

A large pinch sea salt

2-3 teaspoons pumpkin flavored stevia

Method:

1. Add all the ingredients to a blender and blend until smooth.
2. Transfer into a freezable bowl and freeze until done or pour into an ice cream machine and use according to instructions of the manufacturer.
3. Scoop into bowls and serve.

Citrus Pomegranate Fruit Salad

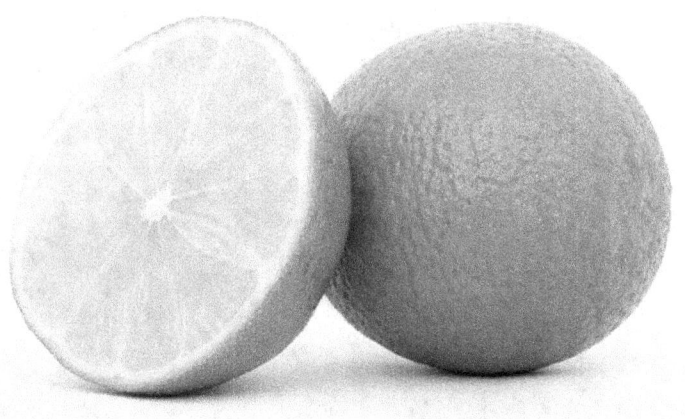

Ingredients:

3 blood oranges, peeled, deseeded, separated into segments

3 oranges, peeled, deseeded, separated into segments

3 pink grapefruits, peeled, deseeded, separated into segments

3 tablespoons raw honey (optional)

1 cup pomegranate seeds

2 tablespoons fresh mint, chopped

4 tablespoons fresh lime juice

Method:

1. Chop the oranges and grapefruit into bite size pieces. Transfer into a large bowl.
2. Add pomegranate, lime juice and honey and mix well. Sprinkle mint.
3. Place in the refrigerator for a few hours to chill.
4. Serve.

Coconut Banana Foster

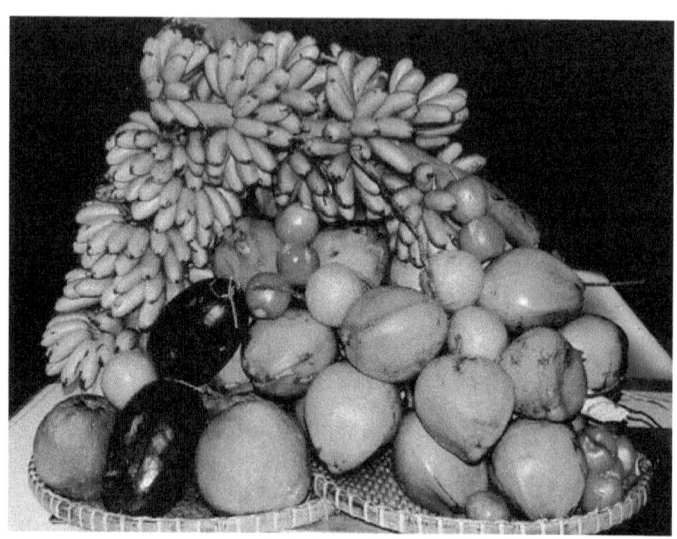

Ingredients:

8 bananas, quartered

¾ cup walnuts, chopped

1 ½ cup coconut flakes

1 ½ teaspoons cinnamon powder

6 tablespoons honey

¾ cup coconut oil, melted

3 teaspoons lemon zest, grated

6 tablespoons lemon juice

1 ½ teaspoon vanilla extract

Coconut cream for serving

Method:

1. Place the bananas in the crock-pot.
2. Sprinkle the bananas with walnuts and coconut flakes.
3. Mix together in a bowl cinnamon powder, honey, coconut oil, lemon zest, lemon juice and vanilla extract. Pour this mixture over the bananas.
4. Set the cooker on Low for 1 ½ to 2 hours depending on how you like the consistency of the bananas to be.
5. To serve, transfer on to individual serving plates. Pour some coconut cream on top of the bananas and serve.

Healthy Sundae

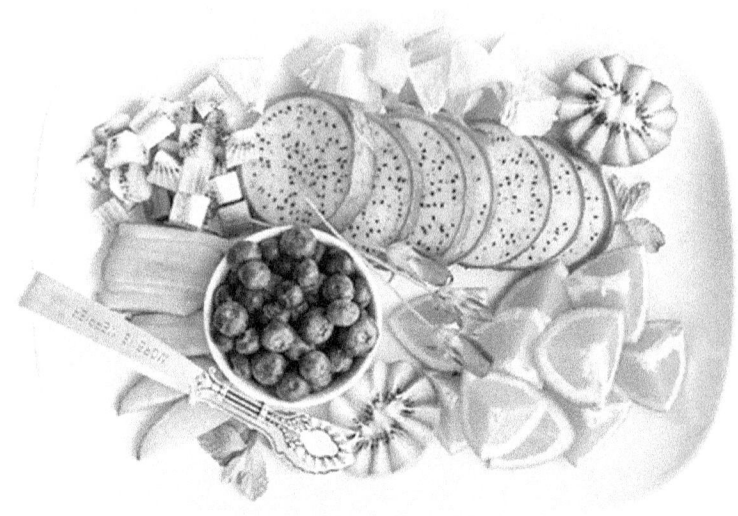

Ingredients:

2 ripe bananas, sliced

2/3 cup pineapple, chopped

2/3 cup kiwi, chopped

4 strawberries, chopped

4 dates, pitted, chopped

¼ cup nuts of your choice

1/3 cup boiling water

1/4 cup almond milk

¼ teaspoon ground ginger

½ tablespoon almond butter, unsweetened

Method:

1. Soak dates in boiling water for at least 45 minutes.

2. Place banana slices on a baking sheet that is lined with parchment paper. Do not overlap the banana slices. Place the baking sheet in the freezer until the slices are frozen.

3. Meanwhile blend together dates and ginger along with water into a smooth sauce and keep it aside.

4. Clean the blender and blend together the frozen bananas, almond butter and almond milk. Transfer into individual freezer safe bowls and freeze until done.

5. Remove from the freezer and sprinkle pineapple, kiwi and strawberry pieces over it. Sprinkle nuts. Pour date sauce on top and serve.

Paleo Chocolate Mousse

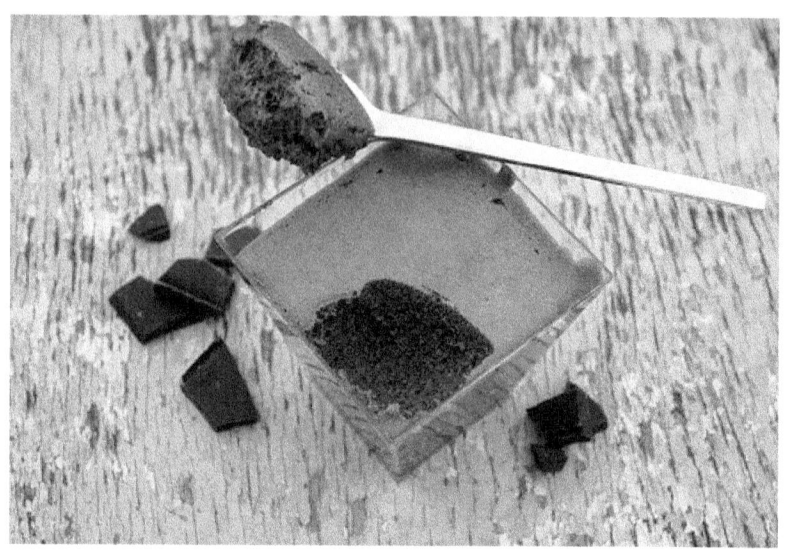

Ingredients:

    2 ripe avocadoes, peeled, pitted, chopped

    2 tablespoons raw honey

    1 cup cacao powder

    ½ teaspoon ancho chili powder

    2 tablespoons pure vanilla extract

    8-10 medjool dates, pitted

    2 cups full fat coconut milk

    2 teaspoons instant coffee powder

    ½ teaspoon Himalayan pink salt

Method:

1. Add avocadoes, dates, coconut milk and honey into a blender and blend until smooth.
2. Add coffee powder, cacao powder (retain a little for garnishing), chili powder, vanilla extract and salt and blend until well combined.
3. Transfer into a mixing bowl. Beat with electric mixer with high setting until the mixture turns light and fluffy.
4. Spoon into dessert bowls. Sprinkle some cacao powder over it.
5. Chill for 5-6 hours and serve

Mixed fruit Cobbler

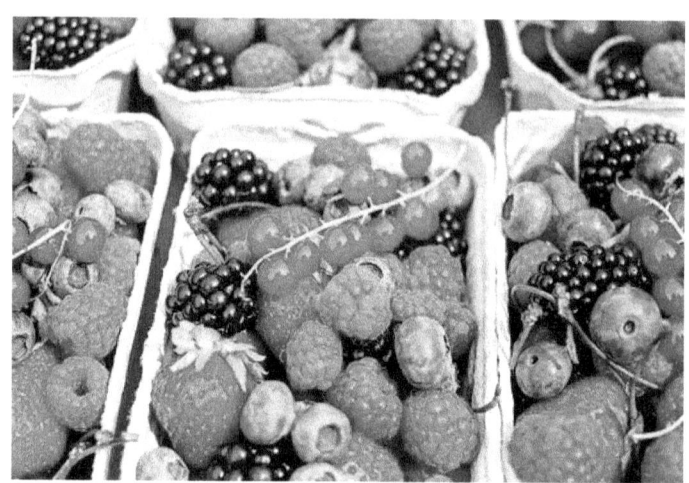

Ingredients:

1 cup frozen strawberries

1 cup frozen blueberries

1 cup frozen raspberries

2 cup frozen peaches

¼ cup coconut sugar

½ tablespoon vanilla extract

2 tablespoons arrowroot powder

For topping:

½ cup almond flour

2 tablespoons coconut flour

¼ cup shredded coconut

2 tablespoons coconut sugar

1 small egg

¼ cup coconut oil

¼ teaspoon ground cinnamon

Method:

1. Place the frozen berries and peach in a large bowl. Leave aside for a while to thaw.
2. When it is not fully thawed, add coconut sugar, vanilla and arrowroot powder and mix well and keep aside.
3. In another bowl, add coconut flour, shredded coconut, coconut sugar and cinnamon. Mix well.
4. In a small bowl, whisk together coconut oil and egg. Add this to the flour mixture. Mix well to get a crumbly texture.
5. Grease a baking dish with coconut oil. Transfer the fruit mixture into the baking dish. Spread the flour mixture over the fruit layer.
6. Place a cookie sheet in the oven. Place the baking dish on the cookie sheet and bake in a preheated oven at 350 degree F for an hour.
7. Remove from the oven. Cool for a while. Tastes best when served warm.

Flourless Peanut Butter Brownie Cookies

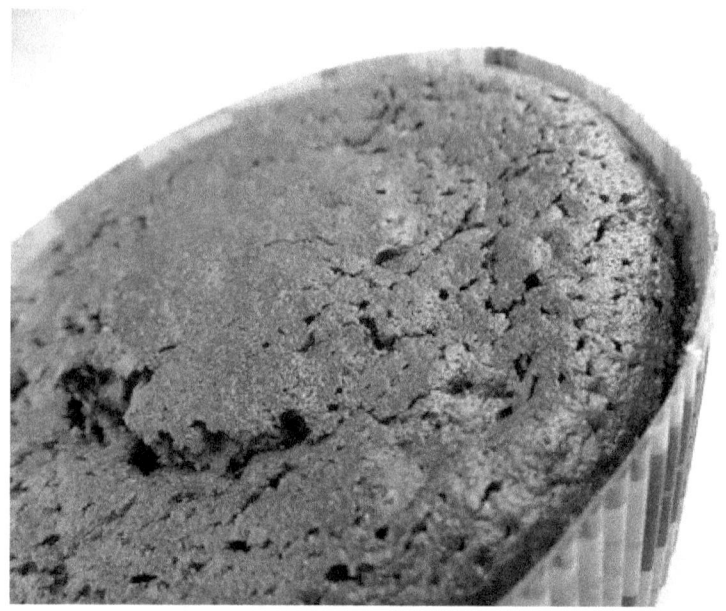

Ingredients:

  2 cups honey roasted peanut butter, at room
  temperature

  2 large eggs

  2 teaspoons baking soda

  1 ½ cups peanut butter chips

  2/3 cup light or dark brown sugar, lightly packed

  1 teaspoon vanilla extract

Method:

1. Line 2 baking sheets with parchment paper.
2. Add eggs into a bowl. Whisk well. Add peanut butter, brown sugar, cocoa powder and baking soda and whisk until well combined.
3. Add vanilla and mix again.
4. Add peanut butter chips and fold until well combined.
5. Drop about 1-½ tablespoons of dough on the baking sheet. Leave space between the cookies. Press the dough (on the baking sheet) lightly with the back of a spoon.
6. Bake in a preheated oven at 4000° F for about 9-12 minutes depending on how crisp you like the cookies to be. Lesser time for softer and longer for crunchier.
7. Store in an airtight container.

Poached Pears

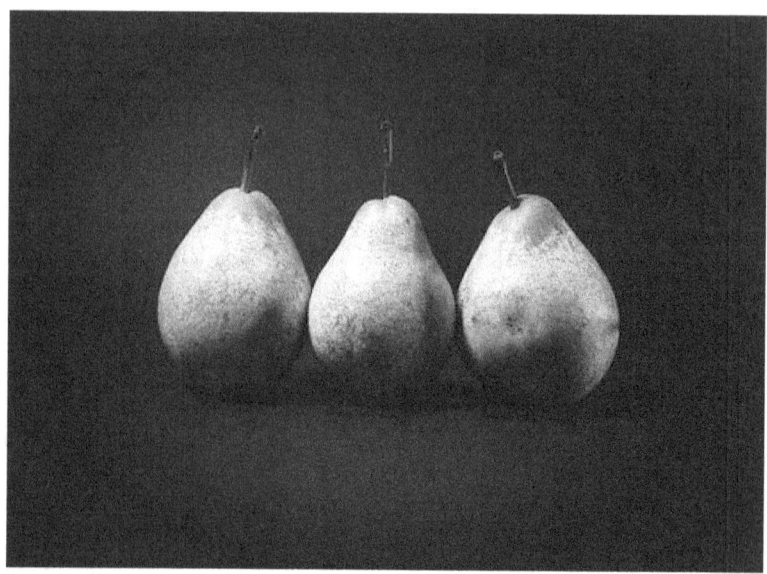

Ingredients:

2 cups coconut sugar

3 tablespoons unsalted butter, chopped into small pieces

8 Bosc pears, peeled, cored, halved

Method:

1. Add coconut sugar, ginger and butter to the crockpot and mix well.
2. Add pears and toss well so as to coat the pears. Place the pears with its cut side on the bottom of the cooker.
3. Cover and cook on High for about 2 hours or the pears are tender.
4. Place a pear in individual bowls. Spoon the caramel sauce over it and serve.

Carrot pudding

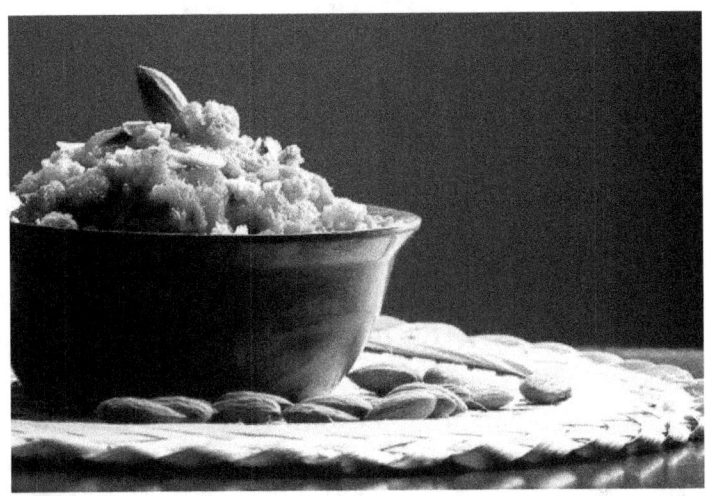

Ingredients:
4 cups carrots, peeled, grated (preferably light red carrots)

2 cups almond milk

Sweetener of your choice like honey, stevia, agave

2 tablespoons raisins

2 tablespoons almonds slivered

2 tablespoons cashews, chopped

½ teaspoon ground cardamom

Method:
1. Place the milk and carrots in a heavy bottomed pan. Place the pan on medium heat. Bring to a boil and simmer for about 15 minutes. Add raisins.
2. Lower heat and simmer until all the moisture is dried up. Stir frequently.
3. Remove from heat. Add almonds, sweetener, cardamom and cashews. Mix well.
4. Serve warm. Left over can be refrigerated. Can store up to a week when refrigerated.

Final Words

Now that you have come to the end of the book, you have a much better idea about the Paleo diet and how it works. The information was put together to help you understand more in a concise manner. We hope it was helpful and reader friendly.

You can see how the diet is a much healthier change from the modern diet that harms our bodies. The foods that are available to us now are very different from what our ancestors ate. Their food was simple and nutritive and definitely did not contain all the harmful additives that we now see in just about everything these days. Follow the lists that we have mentioned to choose what you should include or exclude from your diets. Over time you will see the difference it makes in your body both inside and out. You will see it get leaner and feel more energetic throughout the day.

If you found the information and recipes in this book helpful, you can go ahead and recommend it to any friends or family who could use the push toward a healthier lifestyle as well. Final Words

www.ingramcontent.com/pod-product-compliance
Lightning Source LLC
Chambersburg PA
CBHW062042280526
45788CB00003B/1083